# TABLE OF CONTENTS

# INTRODUCTION

Before my son was born in 2018, I had never heard of exclusive pumping. I was so focused on pregnancy and labour that I didn't spare much thought for what would come after – if I considered it at all, I assumed nursing would be something that would happen easily and naturally.

But my son was born with jaundice. He had to spend 24 hours having phototherapy under a fluorescent light in the special care nursery. He was too tired and lethargic from the jaundice to latch to the breast, so I had to pump to feed him with a bottle and he quickly developed a preference for the bottle over the breast.

Nonetheless, I persevered in trying to nurse. Attempting to get him to latch was stressful for us both – not helped by frequent interruptions from well-meaning visitors. We just didn't have the space and time we needed to work on the problem.

For three weeks I battled to nurse, finally seeking help from a professional Lactation Consultant. She was very confident and explained how she had been able to help thousands of women get their baby back to the breast and it would happen for me too. She then watched me attempt to feed my son. After observing us carefully, she gave me her professional verdict: nothing was wrong. I'd been doing everything right; my son just didn't want to nurse. He simply preferred the bottle.

This left me with two choices; abandon breastfeeding altogether and go to formula or try exclusive pumping.

My partner and I were very keen that our son have the benefits of breastmilk. Since I'd be heading back to work before too long and my partner would be our son's primary carer, I agreed to try it. And so began a gruelling six months of pumping every three hours to express enough milk for my son.

I pumped everywhere; at work, in the car while driving, at home, and out and about. I'd be pumping for 45 minutes at a time, every three hours, even through the night. With few resources available to support exclusive pumpers, I felt alone and exhausted. I'm usually a confident person but being tied to a breast pump all the time felt like I was a cow being milked. It was a big challenge.

We made it to six months, and I remember feeling pride when I saw the freezer stash I had been able to build up, which meant my son was able to continue to have breastmilk for a few weeks longer. But it had been a hard road. I want there to be the resources available for other parents setting out on their exclusively pumping journey, so that you don't feel as alone as I did. Because there are more of us out there feeding our babies this way than you might think.

This book was born from that journey and the desire to put all the information you need about exclusively pumping together in one place. Rather than having to scour the internet for information, I hope this guide will give you all the tips you need, making it simple to discover all the little tricks that make exclusively pumping easier.

I also want you to know that you are not alone, and this does get easier. Once your supply is established and you no longer have to pump during the night, things become less exhausting and overwhelming. Talking about pumping is also so helpful – you learn a lot from other parents who have been on the same journey. Facebook is a great way to find other exclusive pumpers, if you don't know anyone who is doing it in real life.

In 2020, my second child was born during a global pandemic. Although some scary things were going on in the wider world, for us it was a blessing in disguise. Because no visitors were allowed at the hospital, my early days with my new baby were calm and undisturbed. We were able to get nursing established before we left the hospital. Having now done both exclusive breastfeeding and exclusive pumping, I can tell you with certainty that exclusive pumping is ten times harder than nursing. Don't let anyone tell you that you are taking the easy way out!

As mothers, I think we often focus on the negatives and what we've done wrong, or are so focused on the future that we fail to take the time to appreciate our achievements. I've called this book "The Pumping Princess" because in the beginning of my pumping journey, I had never felt less feminine and unattractive in my life. But I now realise, committing to exclusively pumping is an amazing thing and you are a Princess! However far you get on this journey, take a moment to feel pride for everything you have done for your baby.

## Using this guide

The aim of this guide is to cover everything you need to know about exclusive pumping, from making the first decision to pump, to choosing a breast pump, to troubleshooting and weaning. If you are new to pumping or are still pregnant, I highly recommend that you read the book straight through at least once, so that you have all the knowledge you need to be successful.

But I also know what life with a newborn is like, especially when you are stressed about feeding. So this guide is organised into chapters, each with a specific focus. When you need information on a particular issue, you can easily jump into the chapter you need.

After each chapter, there is a quick tips section that summarises the key points in that chapter. When you are in a hurry and need to find information quickly, you can use these sections to prompt your memory, instead of having to read the whole chapter through again.

At the end of the book, you'll find a few suggestions for further reading. While this book aims to be a comprehensive guide with everything you need to know about pumping, there might be times when you are dealing with a very specific issue, or just want to dive deeper into a particular topic. The further reading section will give you some ideas of where to look.

Finally, all the resources used in putting together this guide are in the references section at the end of the book.

Let's get started.

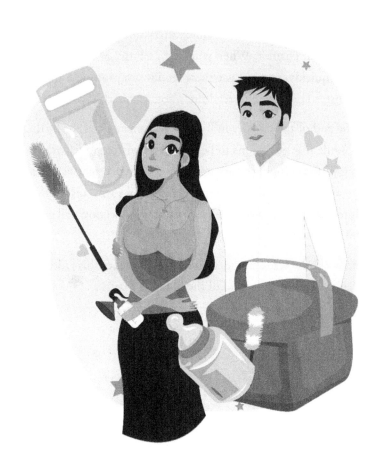

# 1. Getting Started

Whatever your reasons for exclusively pumping, there are a few things you'll need to get yourself started. Researching your chosen method of feeding can help give you confidence and make sure you have the information you need to succeed. That is where this guide comes in – you can find all the key facts about exclusively pumping here and in the following chapters. You can either start by reading straight through, or dip in and out as needed.

Talking to your support network – whether that is a partner, friends, or family members – about exclusively pumping is another good first step. That old saying "it takes a village to raise a child" may be overused but only because it is true. Exclusively pumping to feed your baby will be a key part of your parenting journey in the early months, it is important that anyone supporting you understands what you are doing and how to help.

Finally, the practicalities – having the right equipment is a must. In this chapter, we'll look at both the essentials and the extra kit you might need to make sure your pumping journey goes smoothly. Like anything to do with babies, exclusively pumping can get expensive fast, so concentrate on the essentials first to keep costs under control.

**Deciding to exclusively pump**

You might be considering exclusively pumping to feed your baby before they are even born, or you may have planned to nurse but have encountered problems along the way. Either way, if you are thinking of using this method to feed your child, you are probably already aware of the advantages of breastmilk and want to make sure your baby receives those benefits.

If nursing is off the table, either permanently or temporarily, then exclusively pumping can ensure your baby gets all the immune support, nutrition, and developmental benefits of breastmilk. It does, however, take a bit more time and planning than simply switching to formula. The chapters later in this book on establishing supply and getting into a routine can give you more in-depth information on what is involved. You need to be prepared for multiple pumping sessions a day, particularly in the early months, and unfortunately, breast pumps and bottles mean a lot of washing and sterilising. Having the right equipment can really help in making the whole process as easy as possible.

Discuss your options with your partner, if you have one, as they will be involved with feeding and will, hopefully, be supporting you in finding the time to pump and with the washing and sterilising. If they are worried about the time and effort involved with exclusively pumping, you might want to encourage them to read up on the benefits of breastmilk, so that they understand why you are keen to express milk for your baby.

You could also discuss options with your midwife, child health nurse, or a lactation consultant. Most should be sympathetic to your desire to feed your child breastmilk and will be able to give you advice on how to get started. If you have made the decision to exclusively pump before birth or while still at the hospital, there should be a hospital-grade breast pump available on the maternity ward for you to use once your milk comes in.

## Why choose to exclusively pump?

There are lots of reasons why you might decide to exclusively pump. Whatever your own reasons for choosing this method of feeding, please know that they are valid. Exclusively pumping is often chosen by parents who have had issues with nursing, but this is not always the case. Some reasons you might be interested in exclusive pumping include (but are not limited to);

• Nursing is painful, uncomfortable, or leaves you feeling touched-out

• Your baby has issues with latching or is unable to nurse

• Your baby refuses to nurse

• Your baby is not gaining weight nursing

• You have issues with low supply

• You have issues with oversupply

• Your baby was born prematurely or unwell

• Your baby has allergies or reacts poorly to breast milk at times

• Your gender identity makes nursing a challenge

• You have been nursing, but your baby has started to bite

• You are returning to work or will be separated from your baby for long periods

• You simply prefer to pump rather than to nurse

In any of these cases, or whatever scenario fits your situation, choosing to exclusively pump means that your baby will still benefit from all the health advantages of receiving your breastmilk. Other advantages of choosing to feed this way are that your partner or other caregivers can play an active part in feeding your child, you know how much your baby is drinking, and you can more easily spot patterns with supply in order to troubleshoot if necessary.

## Arm yourself with information

Too often, advice on infant feeding focuses on only two options – nursing and formula feeding. Although the community around exclusively pumping is growing, it is still a neglected area and there is less advice out there for new parents than there should be. This guide will give you all the essential information that you need, and the last section has suggestions for further reading, advice, and support.

The more you know about pumping, establishing your supply, and getting into a routine, the more likely you are to find success and keep up your pumping journey for as long as it suits you and your family.

It can be helpful to share what you learn with your partner if you have one, or anyone else who will be helping you care for your baby in the first year. This ensures everyone is on the same page and understands how exclusively pumping works. One of the advantages to pumping is that your partner or other carers can take a full role in feeding your baby, which can help in creating a strong bond and taking part of the burden off you, while still bringing all the benefits of breastmilk to your child.

## Only you know your family

There are wonderfully supportive communities out there who can help you in your journey as a new parent. But, sadly, becoming a parent can also come with a side-order of judgement. And, for some reason, a lot of this judgement seems to focus on how we feed our children. Sometimes it feels like everyone has an opinion to share, from news outlets to online forums, to that nosy person in the street. Everyone thinks they know best how you should be feeding your child.

Here is the thing – none of those people knows your unique situation as you do, and none of them can choose what is right for your family. That is solely down to you and your partner.

You made the decision to exclusively pump to feed your child for good reasons, and those reasons are valid, no matter what they are. So, once you have decided that this is the route you want to take, trust yourself. Gather the information, equipment, and support you need to make the journey as smooth as possible. Then do your best to filter out all that well-meaning noise from other people so you can concentrate on caring for your baby, and yourself.

There are loads of people who have fed their babies very successfully through exclusively pumping. The chapter on finding support at the end of this book has some suggestions for finding communities, whether in real life or online, who can share their stories, give you tips, and allow you to vent when needed. Knowing you are not alone can be a real comfort, especially on those days when it all feels too much.

## Pumping equipment – the essentials

The good news is that you can get started on your exclusive pumping journey with relatively little equipment, although you might want to add more items later to make the experience more comfortable and less hassle. These are the items that are essential to safe and successful feeding:

## A breast pump

Number one on the list, for obvious reasons, is a good breast pump. In fact, this bit of kit is so essential and there are so many different options, that it deserves a section all its own. Skip to the next chapter for a thorough look at choosing a pump, what to consider, and some of the current options on the market.

## Bottles and bottle teats

Ideally, choose bottles that fit with your pump, which means you can express milk straight into the bottle and saves on washing up. Babies can be picky though, and not every baby will drink from every bottle, so before you buy loads of a single type, make sure your baby will accept the style you have chosen. Some pumps can fit with a range of different bottles, or you can express into a collection bag or the collection unit that came with the pump, then transfer the milk into a bottle for feeding.

Once you have found a style of bottle that suits your baby, you will need at least six bottles. If you have the budget and storage space, buying even more bottles is best to make sure you have enough to cover all your baby's feeds and minimise on how many times you need to wash and sterilise throughout the day. Most styles come in smaller sizes for new-borns and larger sizes for older babies. You can often find multi-packs, which are a less expensive way to buy bottles than single options.

It is worth knowing that bottle teats come in different sizes too. The size you need depends on the age of your baby. Brands can vary, but most label teat size by number and commonly go from 1 to 3. The size of the teat effects the rate of the milk flow from the bottle, so you want the slowest flow for a new-born. The shape of the teat also matters, with most modern bottles designed to limit the amount of air the baby takes in with their milk. This is thought to reduce digestive issues and colic.

## Something to sterilise equipment in

Bottles, teats, and pump parts need to be sanitised at least once a day so that they are safe to use to feed your baby. There is more information on doing this in the chapter on cleaning your pump. While you don't necessarily need a dedicated steriliser for this task if you opt for boiling water or cold water sterilisation, you will need to make sure you have a container big enough to hold everything you want to sterilise in one go. The alternative is to buy a steam steriliser – either an electric one that heats the water itself or one that goes in the microwave.

## Bottle brush and washing tub

If you have a dishwasher and plan on using that exclusively to clean bottles and pump parts, you might be able to skip these, but most people will want them anyway for hand-washing in an emergency. Having a dedicated bottle brush and tub for washing prevents cross-contamination with the rest of the household's washing up, making sure it is safe for your baby. If you are returning to work and plan to wash your pumping equipment there, you can get collapsible washing up tubs which are easier to transport. These can also be useful for holidays and other travel with your baby.

## Milk storage

Especially if you hope to build a freezer stash, having something to store your breastmilk in is essential. There are breastmilk storage bags available which are designed particularly for this purpose – the Lansinoh ones seem to be the most popular, but other brands are available too. Generally, these will have a double zipper to ensure they are leak-proof and can be stored either lying down or standing up, saving you space in the fridge or freezer. They also have gauges marked on them so you can see how much milk is in each one, and space to label them with the date so that you know how long they have been stored for. They are convenient because they come pre-sterilised, so you can use them straight from the pack. But they can be expensive, especially when you are using so many – regular freezer bags can also work.

If you are trying to cut down on single-use plastic, these storage bags might not be the best option for your family. You can, in theory, use any BPA-free container that has an air-tight lid for milk storage, although they will require washing and sterilising before use. There are also reusable options available that are designed especially for milk storage. These are generally small tubs that stack to save space. Once you are done using them for milk, these tubs are useful for storing baby food, toddler snacks, or grown-up leftovers.

### Pumping equipment – additional kit

You can successfully exclusively pump with just the equipment listed above, but there are other bits and pieces that are really useful to have if your budget allows. There's no need to splurge on these all in one go – as you get more established with your pumping, you will have a better idea of which items you might need.

### Extra pump parts

Any part of your breast pump that comes into contact with your milk - that's the breast shield, valves, membranes, connectors, and milk collector bottles or bags – needs to be cleaned and sterilised after every single use. That is a *lot* of cleaning and sterilising, especially when you are pumping 8 to 12 times a day.

This is why most exclusively pumping parents will opt to have several spares of each of these parts. Although not essential, having spare pump parts makes a big difference to the hassle involved in preparing for a pumping session, so this goes to the top of the list for extra kit. It can be difficult to find replacement parts in the shop, but they can usually be bought online, either directly from the manufacturer or via online retailers such as Amazon.

### Hands-free bra

Unless you have a hands-free pump (see next chapter), a hands-free bra can be revolutionary. Without one, you will need to hold the breast shields of your pump in place with your hands, which limits how much you can do while pumping. When you are pumping for two hours or more a day, being able to use your hands makes a big difference, especially if you're a single parent or your partner is out at work.

Hands-free bras vary in style and cost. Some are nursing bras which either have an attachment or have extra fabric panels that hold up the breast shields – these can be worn all day just like a regular nursing bra. Others are a zip-up corset-style affair which goes over your nursing bra and clothes, and which you wear only when pumping. Finally, there are hands-free bands, which aren't bras at all, but instead a kind of harness that goes around your neck and has loops at each end. These loops go around the narrow part of the breast shields to hold them in place. Again, the bands can go over your clothes and nursing bra, although they can be a bit fiddly to position correctly.

Inexpensive hands-free bras of many different styles can be found online on sites like eBay, so there is no need to shell out a lot of money. Like extra pump parts, hands-free bras are not essential, strictly speaking, but the difference it can make to your pumping journey is so great that they are worth investing in.

You can also DIY a hands-free bra, which is a cost-effective option, especially if you are unsure how long you will be exclusively pumping for. You can use a regular sports bra for this and the only additional equipment you need is a pair of scissors. Make sure the bra you choose is comfortable but not so stretchy that it will allow the breast shields to pull away from your breasts once the collector bottle has begun to fill with milk. Cut holes in the bra over where your nipples are (not while you are wearing it though! Use a pen to mark where to cut). You want the holes to be only just large enough to fit the narrow part of the breast shield through. When it is time to pump, you insert the breast shields inside the sports bra and then connect them to your pump through the hole.

## Milk Collectors

Every drop of breastmilk is precious when you are exclusively pumping. Milk collectors catch excess milk that leaks from your breasts so that you can use it later to feed your baby. You can get shell ones, which just sit inside your bra (instead of a breast pad), or larger ones like those made by Haakaa, which also double as a manual pump. These are especially useful for in the shower – the warm water can often stimulate your let-down – and are good for clearing blocked ducts.

If you use a milk collector, it is important to make sure to mix any milk you collect with a pumped feed before giving it to your baby. This is because leaked milk is made up of the thinner foremilk and won't include the thicker hindmilk that you get towards the end of a pumping session. A lot of foremilk on its own can cause lactose overload in your baby because of its high lactose content. This can result in an extremely uncomfortable baby.

## Lactation massager

Lactation massagers are small, handheld massagers that are used to clear blocked milk ducts, ease the discomfort of engorged breasts, and help increase milk supply. There are both manual and battery-powered options available. Although you can simply massage your breasts by hand, a lactation massager is a nice tool to assist and can be more efficient than massaging by hand. If you are thinking of buying a Haakaa hand pump (see above), you can sometimes find offers that include their lactation massager as a package deal. You don't necessarily need to choose a massager that is specifically designed for pumping, but the advantage of many of these is that they are designed to be portable and can often be charged from a USB port.

## Cooler bag

This is especially useful if you are going to be out and about a lot or pumping at work. You'll often find that starter bottle sets, or sometimes even change bags, will come with an insulated bottle holder, but these only hold one bottle, so a cooler bag is really useful for keeping larger amounts of milk cool on the go. It doesn't have to be one made specifically for carrying bottles but look for something that is well insulated and large enough to hold at least 6 bottles, plus ice packs, but not so huge that it is going to be a pain to carry. Babies come with enough equipment as it is!

## Breast pads

Especially early on, you will likely find that your breasts leak quite a bit. Breast pads are circular pads that you wear inside your bra – they absorb any leaks and save you from having to change your shirt every time. You can get both disposable and washable option – there's a bit more of an initial cost for the washable ones, but they save money in the long run, plus are more environmentally friendly than disposables.

## Nursing cover

Not just for nursing, covers can be useful if you want to pump out and about and prefer not to have everything on display. You can easily use a towel or scarf for the same purpose, or a t-shirt loose to cover the pump, but the advantage of a nursing cover is that it allows you to look down the wide neck to check the positioning of your pump or the fullness of your collection bottle.

## Nursing pillow

Those half-doughnut shaped nursing pillows can be useful for bottle feeding too, especially if you plan to pump at the same time as feeding your baby. It gives you somewhere to place the baby that doesn't require you to hold them and the bottle and try to pump, all at the same time. Even with a hands-free pump or bra, there are only so many things one person can manage.

# QUICK TIPS FROM CHAPTER 1

## Deciding to exclusively pump

- Research your options

- Speak to your partner

- Speak to your healthcare provider, midwife or a lactation consultant

- Gather your support network

- Arm yourself with information

- Trust your decision

- Find your community

## Essential equipment

- A good breast pump

- Bottles for feeding

- A way to sterilise pump parts and bottles

- Bottle brush and small washing up tub

- Bags or small containers for milk storage

## Additional kit

- Extra pump parts

- Hands-free bras (or DIY'd sports bras)

- Milk collectors

- Lactation massager

- Cooler bags

- Breast pads

- Nursing / pumping cover
- Nursing / feeding pillow

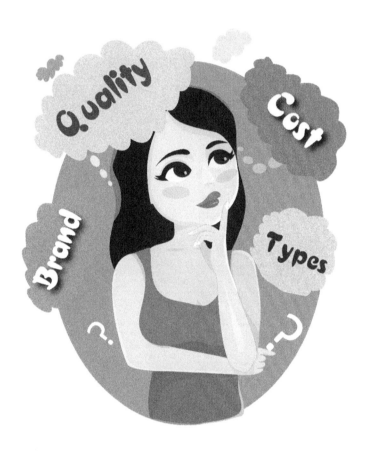

# 2. CHOOSING A BREAST PUMP

There are a lot of different breast pumps out there and finding one that suits you is an important part of setting yourself up for a successful exclusively pumping journey. You are going to be spending a lot of time with this piece of kit. Breast pumps are not a cheap item, although there are ways to cut costs if you are on a strict budget. Even if you are not, it is worth carefully considering the features that are most important to you before making your choice.

The good news is that you don't necessarily need to commit to buying straight away. Hospitals have breast pumps available for use while you are on the maternity ward, and there are hire schemes available to tide you over while you research.

Since choosing a breast pump is so key to exclusive pumping, this chapter includes specific details of some of the different brands and models currently available. The information was compiled in October 2020. It doesn't cover every option out there but does give you an overview of the models most popular with exclusively pumping families.

A further note on cost – this is one area where it makes sense to splash out if you can. Cheap breast pumps rarely have the efficiency and reliability that you need if you are exclusively pumping. It is worth investing a little more to get a pump that works well and has additional features to make your life easier.

## Parts of a pump

Traditional pumps are made up of a pump motor, tube connecting the motor to the milk collection parts, and the collection parts themselves. The collection parts generally include:

- the breast shield (or flange), which is the part that goes over your nipple. Sometimes these will include a removable soft silicone insert that provides cushioning between the shield and your breast

- a back-flow protector that prevents the expressed milk from getting into the tubes and motor

- valves and membranes, which control the suction

- a diaphragm and diaphragm cap, which connect the tube to the collection parts

- a milk collector bottle

## Types of pump

Manual vs electric, single vs double, closed system vs open – there seem to be endless variations of breast pump available. Let's have a look at the differences and which are best for exclusive pumping.

## Manual vs electric

Manual pumps are those that are operated by hand, while electric pumps are powered by a battery pack or connected to the mains. Manual pumps are much less expensive but are not suitable as the main pump for anyone planning on exclusively pumping. They are less efficient than the electric versions, and if you are needing to pump eight times a day or more, they can quickly give you painfully cramped hands.

Having said that, it can sometimes be useful to have a manual pump as a back-up option, just in case you need to express and something has happened to your main pump, such as a broken part, power outage, or flat batteries. Because they are not electric, you can use them in the shower, which may assist with clearing blocked ducts. They may also be useful when you are weaning off the pump at the end of your pumping journey, as a quick way to relieve engorgement.

If you do decide to purchase a manual pump as a back-up, the Haakaa manual pump, mentioned in the last chapter, can double up as a milk collector and is an inexpensive option. Plus, it is made by a family-owned brand based in New Zealand, and is easy to clean, as it has fewer individual parts than many other options. The Medela Harmony and Philips Avent Comfort are two other popular manual pumps to consider.

Electric pumps can come with or without a battery pack. Often models with both are slightly more expensive than those that only have a mains option, but they do allow you to pump on the go. For those without a battery option, it is possible to get a separate battery pack – just be sure to get one the right voltage to work with your pump. You can also get car adaptor chargers for some pumps that allow you to run it while in the car.

As a rule, the pump's suction will be stronger when the pump is on mains power than when it is running off the battery.

## Single vs double

Manual pumps are always single pumps since trying to manually pump both breasts at once really would be a feat. Electric pumps, though, come in either single or double. As the names suggest, single pumps have one breast shield, while double pumps have two.

Double pumps are more expensive but allow you to express milk from both breasts at the same time, which halves the amount of time you need to spend pumping at each session. As a result, they are the best choice for exclusively pumping parents, who are already needing to spend a lot of time pumping every day.

## Open vs closed systems

This is where it gets a little more technical. Open system breast pumps are those that have no barrier between the parts used to collect the milk and the pump system itself. Closed system pumps do have a barrier, which prevents milk from getting into the tubes or motor of the pump. Milk caught in the pump's tubes can go mouldy if you don't notice it in time, so you need to keep a careful eye out if using an open system. Clean and sterilise the tubes if you notice any moisture in them. Milk can also go mouldy if it gets into the motor, which can be a real problem as it isn't possible to clean the motor. Milk contamination is rare, but when you are exclusively pumping it can give you more peace of mind to opt for a closed system.

Closed system pumps tend to be slightly more expensive than open systems. The clinical hospital-grade pumps used on the maternity ward are always closed system pumps. Open system pumps are only suitable for use by one person, so if you are considering a second-hand pump, you will want to go for a closed system one.

## What to look for

So, we've established that the best pumps for exclusive pumping are closed system, double electric pumps. That still leaves quite a wide range of different options. To narrow it down, you need to consider your lifestyle, where you will be pumping most, your budget, and how old your baby is.

## Mobility

Exclusively pumping makes it quite likely that you are going to be pumping on the go, so the mobility of your pump is important. Pumps that aren't too bulky and heavy are best, and those that have a built-in battery pack may be more convenient than those without. Even when you are pumping at home, it is good to have the option not to be tied to a power outlet for every pump session.

## Suction

Suction is also important – the better the suction a pump has, the more efficiently it will empty your breasts and the more milk you are likely to express in a pumping session. Sometimes there is a trade-off between mobility and suction so, if you have the budget, you might consider getting two pumps – one to be your main one for home, and the other for easy use out and about.

Most pumps will come with different suction settings, which allows you to find the level which works best for you.

## Clinical hospital-grade?

The age of your baby and how established your breast milk supply is also plays a part. For new-borns, it is often recommended to use a clinical hospital-grade pump for the first few weeks, as these are the most efficient models. Clinical pumps are the most expensive option though, so you will most likely choose to rent, rather than buy, one of these. You can then switch to a less powerful model once your milk supply is well established and you are in a routine with your pumping. Many people manage just fine without going for a hospital-grade pump though, so if you are on a budget, or already have an established supply, you probably want to skip this step.

## Replacement parts

You also want to consider how easy it is to get replacement parts for the model of pump you choose. Valves and membranes especially need to be replaced often for the pump to work efficiently. Check that you will easily be able to buy replacements and that they won't be too expensive. As discussed in the chapter on getting started, buying some spare pump parts straight away can also make your pumping experience much smoother. Both Amazon and eBay carry replacement parts for many brands of pump, and you can also buy replacements directly from the manufacturer.

## Hands-free

For ultimate ease in pumping-on-the-go, a new generation of pumps is emerging that are designed to be hands-free and discreet, fitting underneath your clothes so that you can pump in public without needing a hands-free bra. They generally have a slightly smaller collection capacity than the traditional bottle collection pumps, but they allow you to be fully mobile while pumping, making expressing sessions less of a chore. They can, however, be expensive, although they arguably save you a bit on buying hands-free bras, so weigh that up in your decision making.

## Size

The breast shield of your pump must be sized correctly to avoid nipple damage and make sure your pump is emptying your breast efficiently. Most manufacturers offer sizing guidance on their websites, so make sure you read these before ordering. You will need to know the size of your nipple (just the nipple itself, not the areola around it). Check that the brand you are interested in offers breast shields of the correct size for you or is compatible with other breast shields if it does not. Pumpin Pals are one option for alternative breast shields if your chosen model doesn't have the right size for you – they have shields of different sizes which are compatible with Medela, Lansinoh, Hygeia, Spectra, Ameda Mya, and Motif Luna.

## Good Pumps for exclusive pumping

This shortlist was compiled in October 2020, so it is worth researching to make sure this advice is still up to date. Prices especially can change. All ballpark prices given here are in Australian dollars. All the pumps on this list are double electric pumps.

## Freemies

Freemie Liberty pumps are a closed system, hands-free option that goes inside your bra. The motor can be clipped to your belt or carried in a bag, so it allows for complete mobility. It has hospital-grade suction and can be charged via a USB port. Shields of different sizes are available and replacement parts can be purchased directly from the manufacturer. Currently, it comes in at around the $400 mark if you buy direct from the manufacturer, but payment plans are available, so you can split the cost across four payments. Note though that the user manual defines normal use of the Freemie Liberty as being three 20-minute pumping sessions a day, which is less than you would expect to be doing when exclusively pumping. Reviews suggest that plenty of parents have successfully used it for exclusive pumping though. Freemie collection cups are also compatible with some other makes of pump, including Spectra, Medela and Ameda.

I had Freemie cups and I connected them to my Spectra S1 and it was extremely useful for hands-free pumping at home. The cups easily inserted into my regular bra.

## Spectra S1 & S2

Very popular amongst exclusively pumping families, the main difference between these two models is that the S1 comes with a rechargeable battery (and is slightly more expensive). These are closed system, hospital-grade pumps known for their quietness and ease of use. The pump unit is light and has a handle so it can be easily moved around, although it is bulkier than other models. They come with a built-in timer, which is helpful for timing pump sessions, and a range of suction settings. There is a dedicated Australian site which includes replacement parts. The S2 comes in at around $300, while the slightly more expensive S1 model is around $380, still making it one of the most affordable high-powered double pump options on the market. Both models are designed for heavy use.

The Spectra S1 was my main pump and the best one I tried, so I can personally recommend it.

## Medela Freestyle and Swing

Medela is one of the most recognisable names in the breast pump world and their clinical Symphony model is used in many hospitals, although it is too costly for home use for most people. The Freestyle is a powerful closed system pump – the newest version, the Flex, has a USB rechargeable battery. It is light and portable and links to an app that can help you track your pumping progress. It is expensive though, at around $550.

The Medela Swing Extra is their less expensive double pump, although it still comes in around the same as the Freemie at $400. Although it too is a closed-system and offers the same level of suction as the Freestyle, it apparently is only designed for use around 4 times a day, which likely won't meet the needs of most exclusively pumping parents, especially in the early days. The Freestyle is designed for heavier use. In both cases, replacement parts are easy to find online.

## Ardo Calypso Double

This closed system pump is recommended by the Australian Breastfeeding Association for exclusive pumpers as an alternative to the expensive hospital-grade Carum model. It is a closed system pump with a wide range of suction settings. It can be run on batteries but is not rechargeable, and batteries must be removed when using it on the mains outlet. In price it is similar to the Medela Swing Extra or the Freemie Liberty, coming in at just under $400.

## Ameda Purely Yours Ultra

The other double pump recommended by the Australian Breastfeeding Association for exclusive pumping is the Ameda Purely Yours Ultra. Again, it is a closed system pump, but this one does not offer a battery option, so you'd need to purchase an external battery pack to make it portable. The price is the most attractive thing about this model – at just $230, it is the most affordable on this list. The sacrifice in portability counts heavily against it, however.

## Hiring a pump

If you are struggling to establish a good supply in the early weeks, hiring a clinical hospital-grade breast pump can be an option to get you started. The Australian Breastfeeding Association offers both the Ardo Carum and the Ameda Platinum pumps for hire at a weekly rate – members get 50% off. You do need to purchase the milk collection kit, however, so make sure that whatever you buy will work with both your hired pump and the pump you ultimately move onto or you may end up having to buy everything again before the parts need replacing. Some chemists will also offer pumps for hire.

Hiring only works out as a cost-effective option for short term use, or for when you need access to one of the clinical hospital-grade pumps that are prohibitively expensive to buy (and overkill for the longer-term needs of most exclusively pumping families).

## Buying Second Hand

Buying second hand might not be an ideal option for everyone. It depends on how comfortable you are buying a pump that has already been used by someone else. But if you are on a strict budget, buying a second-hand pump might mean you can afford a higher-spec model than you could purchase new. Good sites to find second-hand pumps include eBay and Facebook. It is also worth asking around local parenting groups.

Open system pumps are not suitable for buying second-hand, so look for a closed pump system, ideally one of the options listed above that work well for exclusive pumping. On occasion, you can find second-hand pumps that have never been used at all, but if the pump you buy *has* been used previously, you will want to purchase the milk collection parts new to ensure they are safe. That's the breast shields, valves, membranes, backflow protector, and collection bottles.

Ask the seller about the level of use the pump has had previously – since you will be making heavy use of it, it is best to look for a pump that has only been used occasionally in the past, or you risk it breaking or losing suction. If the pump is still within warranty, it is worth researching whether the warranty can be transferred to a new owner – Spectra will allow you to do this with their pumps, making them a good second-hand option.

## Types of pump

• Electric pumps are much better than manual for exclusive pumping, but you may want an inexpensive manual pump as a back-up

• Choose a double pump over a single one for efficient pumping

• Closed system pumps are preferable to open systems, as they are more hygienic and prevent milk from getting into the tubes or motor

## What to look for

• Mobility – portable, battery-powered pumps fit better with exclusive pumping, giving you the freedom to pump out and about

• Suction – for exclusive pumping, good suction and a wide range of suction settings make for more efficient pumping

• Clinical hospital-grade pumps are the most expensive, but useful for establishing good supply in the early weeks. Look to hire rather than buying.

• Replacement parts – make sure spare parts are available and not too expensive

• Hands-free – for pumping in public, specially designed hands-free pumps are the most convenient

• Size – smaller, lighter pumps are less of a pain to carry when pumping outside your home

## Good pumps

• Freemie Liberty – best for convenient, hands-free pumping

• Spectra S1 or S2 – best workhorse pumps, good value for money

- Medela Freestyle – well-established, very popular brand, good for heavy use

- Medela Swing – a more affordable option from this popular brand

- Ardo Calypso Double – recommended by the Australian Breastfeeding Association

- Ameda Purely Yours Ultra – most affordable

## Hiring a clinical, hospital-grade pump

- For establishing supply in the early weeks, but not affordable for long-term use

- Available via the Australian Breastfeeding Association or local chemists

- Purchase milk collection parts separately

## Buying second-hand

- Look for closed system pumps only

- Facebook and eBay can be good sources

- Purchase milk collection parts new

- Ask the seller about previous use

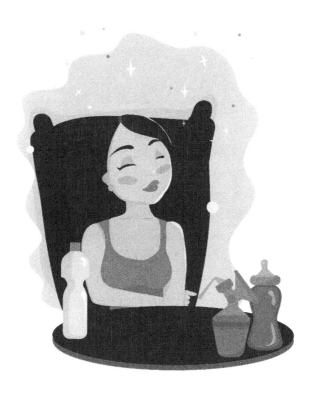

# 3. Using a Pump

Using a pump is a skill and, like any skill, it takes time before you become a true pro. Fortunately, exclusive pumping gives you plenty of time to practice! Before you start, it is always worth reading the user manual for your specific pump, so you know how to assemble it and how to use the different modes and suction strengths. You will also want to clean and sterilise the milk collection parts straight out of the box. If your pump is battery powered, make sure you have charged it before use, or use it on the mains power for the first go.

## Understanding breastmilk

You are most likely to find success in pumping if you know a bit about breastmilk and how the force and make-up of the milk flow changes throughout an expressed feed.

## Colostrum

For the first couple of days after your baby is born, you produce a kind of milk called colostrum, which is very thick and sticky milk that is extremely high in nutrients. Your baby only needs a small amount of colostrum to meet their needs in these first days.

Although you can express colostrum with a pump, the recommendation is to express by hand instead, which seems to work better for this early milk. Hospital maternity wards generally have lactation consultants on hand who can help with your hand expressing technique, and there are also guides and videos available online. It is worth learning this technique anyway as a back-up to pumping but it can take a few tries to get right. You'll only get tiny amounts of colostrum, which is perfectly OK – only a small amount of this wonder milk is needed to keep your baby nourished. A manual Haakaa pump can also work well for colostrum if you are struggling with hand expressing.

## Milk coming in

Around 2-4 days after your baby is born, your milk 'comes in', meaning that the thick colostrum begins to mix with regular breastmilk. This is triggered by the high levels of prolactin present after birth, as well as a sharp drop in progesterone and oestrogen once your baby and placenta have been delivered.

You can usually tell when this has happened, as your breasts will start to feel full and hard, and often start leaking. You will also start being able to express larger amounts, although your baby still won't need loads per feed in the early weeks. Milk supply generally grows over the first 4-6 weeks, as long as you are pumping regularly, and then stabilises. If you have oversupply early on, this often evens out after this initial time as well.

## Foremilk and hindmilk

Covered briefly in the first chapter (under milk collectors), foremilk and hindmilk refer to the changes in milk consistency and fat content during a pumping session. At the start of the session, the foremilk, which is more watery and has a higher lactose content, comes through. Towards the end of the session, the thicker, higher fat, hindmilk appears. You might notice this change in consistency as you pump, especially if you change the collection bottle towards the end of a session. As long as you are fully emptying your breasts during a pumping session, the milk you express will contain both foremilk and hindmilk, but it is not recommended to make a feed up only from collected leaked milk, since this will only contain the foremilk and can cause digestive issues for your baby.

## Letdown

A letdown is when your breasts start to release milk. It usually starts with a fast spray and then settles down into a steady flow of milk. The initial spray can be surprisingly forceful, particularly in the early weeks while your milk supply is getting established, or if you have an issue with oversupply. Most pumps will start in letdown mode, which is a fast, shallow strengthening and release of suction, designed to mimic your baby's initial latch. This stimulates the letdown. Generally, pumps will run in letdown mode for a couple of minutes and then switch automatically to expression mode, which is a deeper, slower suction that encourages the already established flow of milk. You can also toggle between the two modes manually.

After some time, generally 5-10 minutes, the flow of milk slows again to a dribble. The goal when pumping is to stimulate more than one letdown to fully empty your breasts and increase the amount of milk you express in each session.

## Hormones

The two hormones that play a part in producing milk, stimulating letdowns, and establishing an appropriate level of supply are oxytocin and prolactin.

Prolactin, which is produced in the pituitary gland of your brain, is the hormone that tells your body to produce milk. When you pump, the nerves in your breasts send a signal back to your brain that triggers the release of more prolactin. This is why the first advice to anyone struggling with low supply is to pump more, telling your body that more milk is needed. Prolactin is naturally higher at night, which is why middle of the night pumping sessions are important in the later months (more on this in the next chapter).

Oxytocin, often known as the love hormone, is probably a familiar name from antenatal classes, if you took them, because of its role in labour. It is the hormone that stimulates letdown. It is triggered by the letdown mode of your pump, but also by loving and bonding exchanges with your baby. Because of this, you might find having your baby close by while you pump, or looking at pictures or videos of them, helps with getting milk flow started and getting more than one letdown during a pumping session.

**Getting ready to pump**

Especially in the early days, while you are still learning, it is best to find a relaxed and comfortable place to sit while you are pumping, rather than trying to pump while moving around. Once you are more confident, a portable hands-free pump can allow you to multi-task but at the beginning, you are likely to be grateful for the excuse to sit still for a bit.

If your partner or someone else is around, you might want to make them responsible for baby care while you are pumping. If not, and your baby is awake, settle them on your lap or somewhere close by. If you have them on your lap, it is a good idea to have somewhere close where you can safely put your baby down, so you can free up your hands when needed. Babies have terrible timing, so if yours is sleeping when you sit down to pump, don't be surprised if they decide to choose that moment to wake up.

Even with a double pump, sessions are generally 15 to 20 minutes long, so having something to keep you entertained close by can be helpful. Expressing can also make you extremely thirsty and it is a pain to have to interrupt your session to get a drink, so have water or another drink to hand. Hopefully, you have a hands-free bra or hands-free pump to allow you to use your hands but, if not, a straw is useful so you can drink while still holding your pump.

Some pumps have specially angled breast shields that allow you to pump while in a semi-lying down position, which can be the most comfortable, especially if you are recovering from giving birth. If you don't have these, you will need to be in a more upright position to keep the milk flowing into the collection bottle, rather than back onto you. Use cushions and pillows to keep yourself comfortably in position, as it can be a strain on your back otherwise when pumping so often.

Make sure your pump battery is charged or attach your pump to the mains. Anything that comes into contact with the milk should be clean and sterilised before use and you should also wash your hands before you start. If you plan to pour the milk from the pump's collection bottle into another bottle, or storage container, make sure you have that easily accessible.

You might find it helps to give your breasts a massage before you start pumping to stimulate milk production. You can do this by hand or use a lactation massager (see chapter 1).

**Using the pump**

Assemble your pump according to the instructions for your specific model. Make sure that the tubes connecting the collection parts to the motor are firmly on and that valves and membranes are correctly attached. If you don't feel any suction when you turn the pump on, it is most likely because either the tubes have come loose, or the valves are not correctly fitted.

Place the breast shields over your breast, with your nipples at the centre of the openings. Your nipples should be able to move freely in the openings without rubbing against the sides. The breast shields should form a good seal over your breasts, but not feel sharp or uncomfortable.

If you are using a hands-free bra, position the breast shields first before attaching the collection bottles.

Set a timer for the length of time you plan to pump for – some pumps have a timer built-in, or you can use your phone. Start your breast pump in letdown mode. You won't see any milk at first and it can sometimes take a few minutes to start, especially early on. Once letdown occurs and your milk has started to flow freely, switch to expression mode. You can encourage letdown by massaging your breasts as you pump.

Adjust the suction strength in expression mode – a good rule of thumb is to increase the suction until it feels uncomfortable, and then dial it back one. This is the best strength for you. You might feel a tugging or tingling sensation in your nipples, but it shouldn't feel uncomfortable or painful.

Try not to check the collection bottle too often unless it is close to getting full. There's nothing like worrying about the amount of milk you are expressing to make you feel stressed, which in turn slows down your milk production. Chat with a friend or your partner, distract yourself with a book, your phone, a good tv show, or play with your baby.

When the milk flow slows back to a trickle, switch your pump back into letdown mode to encourage a second letdown. You could stop the pump for a moment here to massage your breasts before re-starting. As before, switch the pump into expression mode once you get another letdown.

Pump for the full time you set for the pumping session, even if the milk is no longer flowing (see the chapter on getting into a routine for advice on length of pumping sessions). This tells your body to make more milk and helps to increase your supply.

When you are done, unhook your pump, put the lid on the collection bottle, or transfer the milk to another bottle or storage container, and store it ready for when your baby needs it. Make sure you have a lid secured before you go anywhere with the milk you've expressed, even if you are only taking it to the kitchen. There is nothing worse than working so hard to express a feed and then dropping or knocking over the collection bottle and having it spill everywhere.

# QUICK TIPS FROM CHAPTER 3

## Understanding breastmilk

- Colostrum is the first milk you produce and is best expressed by hand

- After 2-4 days, your normal breastmilk will come in

- Foremilk and hindmilk describe the change in consistency of your milk from the start to the end of a pumping session

- Letdown is when your milk starts to flow. Your pump has two different modes, letdown, and expression. These stimulate letdown

- The hormones prolactin and oxytocin are released by your body and control milk production and letdown

## Getting ready to pump

- Wash your hands

- Clean and assemble your pump

- Make sure batteries are charged, or you are close to a mains outlet

- Find somewhere comfortable

- Decide what to do about your baby

- Have a drink to hand

- Find a way to entertain yourself

- Start with a breast massage

## Using your pump

- Make sure tubes, valves and membranes are correctly attached

- Position breast shields to make sure your nipples can move freely

- Set a timer

- Start your pump in letdown mode

- Switch to expression mode once letdown occurs

- Set the suction level

- Aim for a second letdown

- Keep going for the full time

- Store your milk

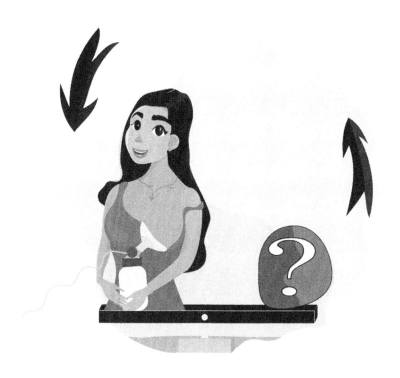

## 4. ESTABLISHING YOUR SUPPLY

In the previous chapter, we looked briefly at colostrum and your milk coming in after birth, as well as the role of hormones in milk production. If you know before you give birth that you are going to be exclusively pumping, the sooner that you start hand expressing after birth the better, as this sends a signal to your body that the colostrum is needed. Once your milk comes in, you will need to pump regularly to establish a good supply of breastmilk for your baby.

In this chapter, we'll look at how your supply changes and regulates within the first 12 weeks after giving birth. We'll also look at issues with supply and how to troubleshoot them.

### Supply in the early days

Once your milk comes in a few days after giving birth, your supply is often all over the place. It hasn't yet settled into a good supply-and-demand routine with your baby's needs. You can encourage your supply to become well-established by pumping regularly – at least 8-12 times a day, mimicking the normal feeding pattern of a new-born baby.

You may not get much milk the first few times you pump, which is completely normal. Not only are you still getting your supply established, but your body is getting used to the pump and you may be tenser than you will be later once you have gained more confidence. While in an ideal world you'd be able to express a full feed, or even slightly more, every time you pump, the reality is that you may not achieve this with every pumping session, especially in the early days.

## Regulation

By the 12-week mark, most people find their supply has regulated. In fact, it generally happens a bit earlier. This means that your supply is no longer being controlled by the drop in oestrogen and progesterone and increase in prolactin from giving birth, but instead by the oxytocin and prolactin produced in response to your pumping sessions. The hormones released by pumping create a supply and demand system that tells your body how much milk is needed to feed your baby.

Once your supply has regulated, you will probably find you have less leakage than in the early weeks. Your breasts won't feel engorged as often, unless you go an especially long time between pumping sessions, and you might notice a dip in supply.

Even once your supply has regulated, there are still things you can try to increase or reduce how much milk you express.

## Supply issues: Undersupply

Undersupply is when you are regularly producing less milk than your baby needs. It is worth noting that expressing smaller amounts than your baby drinks is not necessarily a sign that you aren't producing enough milk. Breast pumps are less efficient at removing milk from the breast than a baby who is nursing well, so it may be an issue with your pump, rather than a supply issue. Before starting to try techniques to boost supply, you might want to try replacing the valves/membranes in your pump, especially if you have been using it for 2 months or more. You can also make sure you are making the most of your pumping sessions by doing breast compressions, using a vibrating lactation massager, putting a warm compress on your breasts, and pumping with your baby close by to encourage the release of oxytocin. All of these can help encourage letdown

If you suspect your issue is more with the amount you express, rather than the amount you produce, you can also try pumping in the shower. Obviously don't take your electric pump into the shower with you, but if you have a manual pump too, the warm water can often help with stimulating letdown. You likely don't want to try this at every pumping session since constantly hopping in and out of the shower is a bit of a task, but it can help to determine whether you are having issues with low supply, or with pumping itself.

If your pump is in good working order and you still need to up the amount of milk you are getting at each pumping session, here are some things to try:

## Pump more often or for longer

The best way to tell your body to produce more milk is to stimulate the release of more prolactin, the hormone that controls breastmilk production. Prolactin release is triggered when your nipples are stimulated during a pumping session, so the more you pump, the more prolactin your brain releases, and the more milk you will produce.

You can either add in extra pumping sessions, pump for longer per session, or both. It will take a couple of days for your body to catch up with the demand for more milk and starts to up production, so don't be discouraged if you get the same amount of milk you were getting with fewer sessions at first.

Watch out for burn out though – there's only so much time you can spend tied to your pump before it becomes too exhausting, especially with a small baby and perhaps other children to care for. Your mental health needs to come first.

## Try power-pumping

New-borns are well-known for cluster feeding, especially in the evenings. Cluster feeding is when a baby wants to feed very often over a period of around two hours or so. The feeds will be shorter than usual. Both bottle-fed and nursing babies cluster feed, usually just before they go through a growth spurt. It seems to be nature's way of telling your body to up the milk production to meet the baby's increased needs.

If you are having issues with low supply, power-pumping is a way of mimicking your baby's cluster feeding behaviour and telling your body to ramp up the amount of milk you are making. It involves grouping together lots of shorter pumping sessions within a period of about an hour. You start by pumping for 20 minutes and then alternate 10 minutes rest and 10 minutes pumping for the rest of the hour. Since you'll be tied to your pump during a power-pumping session, make sure you have drinks, snacks, and entertainment to hand and use a hands-free bra or hands-free pump.

It might help to have someone else be in charge of your baby while you are power-pumping or to try to time it for when your baby sleeps so that you can concentrate on pumping. It is difficult to sit down for an hour if your baby is awake and there is no one else on hand to help. Early evening may be a good time to schedule a session, once your baby and any other young children are in bed.

Aim for one power pumping session a day for between four days and a week. The power pumping session should replace one of your regular pumping sessions.

## Pump at night

Prolactin levels are highest at night, so making sure that you are pumping at least once at night, between 1 am and 4 am, both takes advantage of higher milk production at this time and sends a strong signal to your body to up your supply. You should expect to need to pump at night until at least the 12-week mark. There are some tips in the next chapter for how to make middle of the night pumping sessions less of a chore.

## Stay well hydrated

Producing breastmilk can make you extremely thirsty, your body's way of letting you know if you need to up your liquid intake. But it is easy to become distracted when you are pumping and also caring for a small baby. Keep a drink to hand whenever you sit down to pump to make it easier to get the fluids you need. A portable water bottle can be useful for out and about. It doesn't have to be water if you find that boring, just any hydrating fluid.

Although clinical studies have not found a connection between good hydration and breastmilk supply, anecdotal evidence suggests it can help. Since staying well hydrated is good for your general health, it is worth a try. But don't force yourself to drink if you aren't thirsty – your body knows how much it needs.

## Eat porridge

Like upping your water intake, eating porridge to increase breastmilk supply isn't something that has been clinically proven to work but is another simple and low-cost thing to try. If nothing else, porridge is a nutritious food that contains plenty of iron – low iron levels are common during pregnancy and breastfeeding, so having porridge for breakfast is a good way to address this. Many people, including lactation consultants, recommend porridge to help with low supply.

If you aren't a fan of cooked porridge, look for other ways to incorporate oats into your diet. You can blend them into a smoothie, bake them into lactation biscuits, or toast them with nuts and seeds to make muesli. If making your own oat-based snacks sounds like a chore too far right now, you can also buy mixes and pre-made lactation biscuits online. As well as oats, they include a mix of 'galactagogues' (herbs, foods, or drugs that increase milk production) to help tackle your low supply.

## Other galactagogues

Like the lactation biscuits mentioned above, you can buy specialist tea blends and smoothie or shake powders that contain a mix of galactagogues. Popular herbs include blessed thistle, fenugreek (which has the strange side effect of making you smell like maple syrup), goat's rue, and fennel, all of which can help with milk production. Brewers' yeast is another popular galactagogue but has quite a distinctive flavour that some find off-putting, so is most often found in lactation biscuits or as part of a shake mix. You can also buy it in powdered form to add to smoothies.

The concentration of all of these when found in teas, biscuits and shakes can be fairly low, so if you have tried this route and not had success, you might want to try taking herbs in tablet or capsule form instead. Again, these can be bought online, or from some health food shops or chemists. Fenugreek especially is one that many people swear by for increasing supply but be aware that others have found that it does the opposite and causes a dip instead. You might want to try other methods first just in case.

## Medication

As well as the natural galactagogues discussed above, research has shown that the motion sickness drug Motilium (brand name for domperidone) is effective in increasing levels of prolactin and can therefore make your body produce more milk. It is only available with a prescription so you will need to talk to your doctor if you would like to give it a try.

Many people have reservations about taking medication while expressing milk for their babies. Motilium seems to be safe – very little indeed crosses over into breastmilk so the amount that your baby will get is negligible. It can have some side effects for you though – some people report headaches, dry mouth, or cramps, although most don't experience any problems at all while taking it.

Doctors can vary in their attitude to prescribing Motilium for increasing breastmilk supply – some positively encourage it, while others won't prescribe it at all. If you want to try it, you might first want to go through the other suggestions on this list. You should also keep a log of how much you can pump per day. If your doctor is on the fence about prescribing Motilium, going in with evidence that your supply is indeed low and that you have tried other methods without success might help to convince them. In many ways, one of the advantages of pumping over nursing is that you have a solid idea of how much milk you are able to express per day. You may as well use this evidence to good advantage.

Motilium has been linked to heart arrhythmia in rare cases – usually where it was given in high doses to patients who already had an underlying illness. This shouldn't be a problem but if you have had heart problems in the past, your doctor will likely advise you against taking Motilium.

As well as Motilium, the anti-nausea drug metoclopramide (brand name Apo) is another prescription drug that has been found to be effective in increasing milk production. However, unlike Motilium, Apo can cross the blood-brain barrier and has been linked to side effects such as diarrhoea and depression, so if you are considering medication, Motilium is likely the safer choice.

## Speak to a lactation consultant

If you have tried everything and your supply is still not where it needs to be or you just want some support from a professional, try speaking to a lactation consultant. Many will be more used to working with nursing parents than people who are exclusively pumping, but they will still have helpful advice on managing supply issues. Just be upfront about the fact you are exclusively pumping so they know to offer appropriate advice. A lactation consultant is different from a breastfeeding counsellor, who are usually volunteers. You can find a lactation consultant via LCANZ: Lactation Consultants of Australia and New Zealand: https://www.lcanz.org/find-a-lactation-consultant/

**Supply issues: Oversupply**

Often during the first couple of months, things go the other way, and you find that your body is actually producing more milk than your baby needs. In fact, difficulties with oversupply may be one of the reasons you decided to exclusively pump in the first place – sometimes the letdown can be so strong your baby can't cope with it. Oversupply can also cause the foremilk/hindmilk imbalance issues discussed in the previous chapter, resulting in an upset baby.

It is important not to let oversupply in the early weeks fool you into pumping less often, as this normally doesn't last beyond around the 12-week mark (at the latest). If you haven't been pumping regularly when your supply regulates you may find you are expressing less milk than you need. This is because milk production is no longer controlled by the hormone changes from giving birth, but on a supply and demand basis triggered by how often your breasts are emptied.

If you are pumping more milk than your baby needs, use the extra milk to start a freezer stash, so you can get ahead of your baby's feeds and make sure you have sufficient milk to tide you over if your supply drops a little later, or your baby goes through a growth spurt.

You might see advice on coping with oversupply that tells you not to pump too often for fear of making the issue worst. This is usually more aimed at people who are both nursing and pumping rather than exclusively pumping, but if oversupply is causing you problems with engorgement and painful breasts, is giving your baby digestive issues, or continues past the point when your supply should have regulated, there are some things you can try to address the issue.

### See a lactation consultant

It is a good idea to start by checking in with a lactation consultant if you have issues with oversupply, as they can confirm that you are producing too much and then help you to put a game plan into place to reduce your supply. As mentioned above, you can find a consultant via Lactation Consultants of Australia and New Zealand (LCANZ): https://www.lcanz.org/find-a-lactation-consultant/.

### Reduce the number or length of pumping sessions

It can be difficult to drop a pumping session when you have oversupply, as your breasts quickly become engorged and you run a higher risk of clogged ducts. But you need to tell your body to release less prolactin to reduce your supply. Fewer pumping sessions mean less stimulation of your nipples and therefore less prolactin. If it is too uncomfortable to drop a pumping session altogether, you could instead try to reduce the amount of time you pump for at each session.

Go gradually in both cases – there's more advice on dropping pumping sessions in the next chapter on routines. If you are reducing the length of your pumping sessions instead, shorten them by three or four minutes, wait a couple of days, then shorten again, until you are producing the right amount for your baby's needs. Keep a careful eye on your baby while reducing the length of sessions – you want to make sure you are pumping long enough to get the hindmilk. If they start to have green frothy nappies, that's a sign of foremilk/hindmilk imbalance.

### Reduce the volume of milk you pump per session

Like reducing the number or length of sessions, gradually cutting down on how much milk you pump at each session can signal to your body that it is producing more milk than needed. The difference is that you set a volume goal rather than a time one. So, if you would generally expect to pump 8 ounces at a particular session, stop your pump when you get to 7 ounces instead. This might need you to pay a little more attention than reducing the time spent pumping, as you'll need to keep an eye on your collection bottle. You may want to start with one pumping session at a time to avoid issues, then gradually reduce the volume you pump at other sessions until you get to a happy balance.

## Take a lecithin supplement

Lecithin is found in several different foods, including sunflower seeds, soybeans, and eggs. It is an emulsifier, which means it breaks down fat. If you are experiencing oversupply, taking a lecithin supplement can help prevent clogged ducts, allowing you to go longer between pumping sessions and eventually drop a session more easily. Lecithin supplements are classed as herbal supplements, so you can get them without a prescription, online or from some health food stores or chemists.

## Try cabbage leaves

You might have heard the old wives tale about putting cabbage leaves in your bra to relieve sore leaky breasts. Well, unlike a lot of old-wives tales, this one appears to be true. No one is quite sure why it works, because it hasn't been a huge area of research, but it does seem to. Use two leaves from the inside of a chilled green cabbage, give them a rinse, and then wrap them around your breasts, leaving your nipples uncovered, and secure with your bra. Remove after about half-an-hour. You'll want to do this 2-3 times a day.

## Use herbs

Sage and peppermint are two common herbs that can help with reducing supply. Spearmint, lemon balm, and oregano are also useful. They can be taken as a tea or made into a massage oil for use on your breasts. Some people have also had success with ultra-strong peppermint candies.

## Take birth control pills

Birth control pills containing oestrogen are known for reducing milk supply. Talk to your doctor if you think going onto birth control might help with oversupply issues so they can recommend a suitable option. This one is probably a last resort since if it reduces your supply too far, coming back off the birth control might have side effects during the transitional period.

## Take Sudafed

More commonly known as a decongestant, Sudafed has also been found to permanently reduce milk supply with regular use. It is available without prescription from chemists. Again, use with caution as you don't want to go too far and end up producing less milk than your baby needs.

## What should you do with the excess milk?

If you are ending up with too much milk to store in the freezer, you might want to look into donating it, either to a hospital for use in the NICU or directly to other families that might need it. You could offer it up informally in your local parenting group, or there are dedicated Facebook groups that people use to find donor milk.

If you have older children, you could use some of the breastmilk for them on their breakfast or in a smoothie. Or give your baby a breastmilk bath – this is good for using up milk that has reached its use-by date and can't be safely drunk. Breastmilk baths are great for your baby's skin, especially if they suffer from eczema or nappy rash. You just mix a bag or two of breastmilk with water and let your baby soak.

# QUICK TIPS FROM CHAPTER 4

### Supply in the early days

- Establish supply by pumping every 2-3 hours

- Don't be discouraged if you don't pump much at first

### Regulation

- Supply usually regulates by 12 weeks after birth

- Your breasts will leak less and are less likely to become engorged

- You may find your supply dips

### Undersupply

- Before troubleshooting undersupply, check that your pump is working properly

- Replace pump parts

- Make the most of pumping sessions using breast massage and keep your baby close by

- Try pumping in the shower

- Pump more often or for longer

- Try power pumping

- Stay well-hydrated

- Eat porridge or oats in other forms

- Use galactagogues such as fenugreek, blessed thistle, goat's rue, fennel, and brewers' yeast.

- Consider medication

- Talk to a lactation consultant

## Oversupply

- Some oversupply is common before supply regulates

- Be careful of treating oversupply issues before 12 weeks after birth

- See a lactation consultant

- Reduce the number or length of pumping sessions

- Reduce the volume of milk you pump at each session

- Take a lecithin supplement

- Try cabbage leaves

- Use herbs such as sage, peppermint, spearmint, lemon balm, and oregano

- Go on birth control

## What to do with excess milk

- Donate milk

- Give it to older children

- Give your baby a milk bath

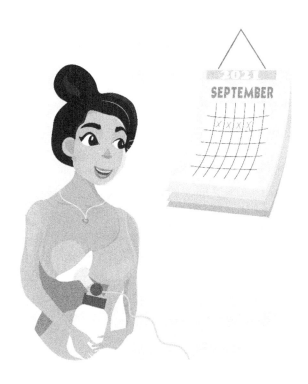

## 5. GETTING INTO A PUMPING ROUTINE

Babies like to keep us on our toes, so the one thing you can guarantee is that you will have just settled into a comfortable routine when they decide to have a growth spurt, go through a sleep regression, or hit a new developmental milestone and you have to start again from scratch. So, when we talk about getting into a routine in this chapter, it is very much about guidelines, rather than hard and fast rules. What works for you will depend on a lot of different factors – your baby's temperament, your own, how much support you have, whether you have older children, whether you work, etc. If what you end up doing looks completely unlike the suggestions in this chapter, it doesn't mean you are doing anything wrong. Finding what works for you and your baby is what matters.

### The first 4-6 weeks

The first 4-6 weeks after giving birth are generally the most intense. By the 6 week mark, you will probably find you have settled into a pumping routine, are comfortable using your breast pump, and have found some ways to manage juggling a new-born with the demands of exclusively pumping. This doesn't mean that issues won't come up from time to time, but it will hopefully all be feeling a little less overwhelming.

During these early weeks, the aim is to pump in a way that mimics the way your new-born would feed if they were nursing. This means pumping every two to three hours during the day, and at least once at night, when levels of prolactin are high. New-borns have small stomachs, so they feed little and often, typically eight to twelve times in 24 hours. You want to mimic this with your pumping routine. Regularly emptying your breasts lets your body know to up your supply to meet demand. Aim for a minimum of two hours pumping per day, split across 8 to 12 sessions.

There are two main ways to organise your pumping sessions. You can either work by the clock, pumping at the same time every day, or follow your baby, timing your pumping sessions for when they feed. The first option might work better for you if you are someone who needs a strong routine. The second option has the advantage of matching your pumping sessions closely to the natural feeding rhythm of your baby.

You can also go for a mixture of the two – keeping to a consistent time for some pumping sessions and following your baby's lead for others. You might, for example, want to pump first thing when you wake up and just before you go to bed, both to ease any discomfort and to get ahead of your baby's feeds. If you are trying to raise your supply through power-pumping, you'll likely need to set aside a specific time to do that, as it is time-consuming.

You will probably find this changes as your baby grows – there is often little set routine in the early months but many babies will fall into a natural schedule as they get older.

Knowing roughly how many pumping sessions you will be doing in 24 hours helps in working out how long to pump for. If you should be aiming for 2 hours a day, and you usually pump 10 times, each pumping session needs to be at least 12 minutes long. You can go for longer – if your milk is still flowing at the 12-minute mark, it doesn't make much sense to stop, unless you are trying to reduce your milk production. But try to pump for the full time even if you are no longer getting any milk so that you establish a good supply.

## How much do newborns eat?

The amount of milk your newborn will eat will vary a bit depending on their size and appetite but on average a newborn will drink 2 to 3 ounces of milk per feed, every two to three hours, with perhaps one longer stretch between feeds at night. Their milk intake will grow for about the first month and then usually stabilises at somewhere around 25 ounces per 24 hours – although, again, this will vary quite a bit dependent on your baby. The amount they drink tends then to stay fairly steady until they start on solids at around 6 months, but they will likely consolidate into larger, less frequent feeds.

If you are trying to work out roughly how much you will need to pump for each feed, divide 25 by the number of feeds your baby has per day – e.g. 25 divided by 9 would be 2.8, so you'd want to aim for 3 ounces per feed. Your baby's hunger might vary across the day – some babies will drink a bit more for their first feed of the morning, for example, so you might want to keep a diary for a few days to see if any patterns emerge that can help you plan how much milk you need. There are apps available that can help you keep track of your pumping sessions and how much your baby eats, which can be very useful during the foggy, sleep-deprived newborn days.

## Middle of the night pumping

Tiring but necessary, pumping in the middle of the night is an important part of establishing your supply in the early weeks. Prolactin levels are higher at night, meaning it is an important time to let your body know to make milk. You also shouldn't go more than 4 or 5 hours at a time between pumping sessions while establishing your supply. Going too long between pumping sessions can lead to clogged ducts, as well as low supply. Plan to pump at least once during the night, between 1 am and 4 am for at least the first 12 weeks (and likely longer if your baby continues to wake during the night to feed). For the first couple of months, you might need to pump twice a night.

It is really, really tempting to skip the middle of the night pumping session when you are already so tired from being up in the night with your baby and caring for them during the day. Resist the temptation, at least in the early weeks, as this session is important for establishing your supply. While nothing is going to make you leap out of bed at 3am excited to pump, there are some things which can make it less of a hassle:

### Prepare in advance

Put together a little basket of supplies – a drink, something to read or do (your phone can be a useful source of entertainment since it comes equipped with a screen light), your pump, and anything else you need for a comfortable pumping session. Make sure your pump is either plugged in or charged in advance and is fully assembled, ready to go. Set everything beside your bed so you don't have to get up to start pumping.

### Don't set an alarm.

This might sound counter-intuitive when we've just discussed the advantages of pumping at night, but your nights with a small baby are going to be disturbed enough without being woken up by your alarm too. Your baby is going to be waking you up anyway during the first few months, so instead of having your alarm wake you while your baby is sleeping (and risk waking them up too), use their cues to let you know when to wake up to pump. This has the added advantage of mimicking their natural feeding pattern with your pumping sessions.

## Share the load

If you have a partner, they can take care of the feeds and nappy changes. Since you are on pumping duty, your partner can be in charge of feeding the baby. When they wake, you can start your pumping session while your partner takes care of the baby's needs. This means you reduce the amount of time you all have to be awake for.

## Multi-task

If you don't have a partner, now is the time to multi-task. If you can manage it, try to pump and feed your baby at the same time. It takes a bit of juggling, especially at first, and you will want either a hands-free pump or the nursing bra style of hands-free bra that you can sleep in. Hopefully, your baby will be able to finish their feed and fall asleep while you finish your pumping session and you can transfer them back to their crib when you are done. Change their nappy before you start the feeding/pumping as they will likely fall asleep during the feed.

## Get a white noise machine

The quietest pump is noisy in the middle of the night and the last thing you want in the middle of a sleep-deprived pumping session is for your pump to disturb your baby. White noise machines help get babies to sleep well anyway and can block out the noise of your pump.

## Buy some angled breast shields

Breast shields that allow you to pump while semi-reclined are ideal for middle of the night pumping sessions. Although you probably want to avoid dropping fully back to sleep while pumping, unless you are a very still sleeper, you can at least prop yourself up on a pillow and doze while you pump.

### Dropping night pumping sessions

Once your supply is well-established and your baby is needing to feed less at night (perhaps just once instead of two or three times), you likely want to drop one of your night-time pumping sessions so that you can get more sleep. The trouble can be that your body has gotten used to producing milk for this nightly session. You may find weaning off a night feed causes problems with engorgement. One option is to slowly move the session later and later rather than dropping it all at once, especially if you are prone to blocked ducts. You can try moving it back half-an-hour each night until it is only an hour before the first feed of the morning, at which point you can drop it altogether. You can also go more slowly if pushing it a whole hour later each night is causing you issues.

If you are impatient to get more sleep and don't typically have issues with clogged ducts, you can try dropping the session all at once instead. If you go this route, you will probably have an uncomfortable couple of nights while your body adjusts, so consider using some of the techniques from the previous chapter under the section on oversupply, such as putting cabbage leaves in your bra or taking a lecithin supplement.

Another option is to try keeping the session at the same time but reducing how long you pump for by a few minutes each night until you are not pumping at all. The problem with this method can be that it is harder to keep track of how long you are pumping for when you are feeling sleepy in the middle of the night – a pump with a timer can help here or you can use the timer on your phone.

Finally, you could try reducing the volume you pump at each session – aiming for an ounce less every night until you drop the session entirely. This one requires a certain degree of concentration, so might not work for you if you prefer to doze during your night-time pumps.

When dropping a night pumping session, keep a careful eye on your supply during the rest of the day. If your supply is well-established, it shouldn't cause issues – you will likely find that your first session of the morning is more productive and makes up some of the difference. But if you are finding that your supply drops too low, you may need to reinstate the feed and keep it going for a few more weeks.

## Adapting as your baby gets older

As your baby grows, so does their stomach, meaning they can take in more milk in one go and wait longer between feeds. Depending on how your pumping sessions are going, as your baby consolidates their feeds, you can do the same with your pumping. As with pumping with for a newb-born, you are aiming to mimic your baby's natural feeding rhythm, so you want to be pumping less often, but for longer each time.

For example, if your baby has been having eight bottles a day and has now gone down to seven), you might have been pumping eight times a day for 15 minutes. You drop one pumping session to match your baby and now want to be pumping for 17 minutes at every session – the time you spend pumping is the same, but it is consolidated into fewer feeds.

Typically, babies settle into roughly a four-hour feeding pattern by around the three to four-month stage, although all babies are different, so if yours is needing to feed more regularly still by this age, don't be surprised. Lots of babies also eat slightly more frequently in the evening, so you might find their last two feeds before bedtime are closer together.

Whether you drop a pumping session every time your baby drops a feed depends a little on what your aims are. If your supply is lower than you would like, you might keep the extra pumping session for a bit longer to encourage your body to produce more milk. You might also want to keep the extra session if you are aiming to build a freezer stash, especially if you will be going back to work soon or are planning to stop pumping but still want your baby to be able to have some breastmilk.

If you do decide to drop a pumping session, the suggestions above for dropping a night feed also work for dropping a session during the day: push the session later, pump for less time, pump less volume, or drop it all at once. Don't forget to add the extra pumping time to your other sessions as you go to avoid a dip in supply.

## Pumping once your baby starts solids

Once your baby is around 6 months old you will start to introduce them to solid food. Initially, this will cause very little change to your pumping schedule, as most babies are still dependent on milk as their main source of nutrients for several months yet. There's an exhausting patch when you first introduce solids when your baby is still having breastmilk five or six times a day, and you are having to pump, and they are having solid food too. During this time it can feel like all you do all day is prepare food (solid or liquid), feed your baby, wash-up, and then start the whole thing over again. Fortunately, it doesn't last too long. Batch cooking baby appropriate meals and delegating the cooking and washing up to your partner can help. Baby-led weaning might also be a good thing to explore, as it involves offering your baby solid food instead of purees right from the start, meaning you don't have to prepare meals especially for your baby.

After a while, solid food will stop being something your baby mainly plays with, or wears, and will start playing a genuine role in their daily diet. As this happens, you will likely notice they are wanting to drink milk less often, or drink less per feed. This is a signal that you can start looking to drop further pumping sessions. By 10-12 months, your baby will probably have three solid meals a day.

## Out and about

In the very early days, pumping while out and about might feel like an impossible task. But as you gain confidence, you are likely to want to be less tied to home, which means you will need to plan how to pump while out and about. Having a hands-free pump like a Freemie can make a huge difference here, as they are designed to be discreet and portable. They can go inside a regular nursing bra and the motor unit can be clipped to your belt, so you can easily pump in public without worrying about privacy, other than when you start and end the session.

If you only have one of the more traditional breast pumps, like a Spectra or Medela, how you handle pumping while out and about depends a bit on your own level of comfort. Expressing milk in public is covered by the Sex Discrimination Act 1984, the same laws that cover nursing. This gives you the right to pump wherever you need to without being discriminated against.

You do not need to cover up unless you want to but, if you do prefer to cover up, a nursing cover can work just as well to hide pumping equipment, or you could wear a loose top or use a scarf, blanket, or towel. Unlike a baby, a breast pump doesn't need to breathe, but it is helpful to be able to check the positioning of your breast shields and the level of milk in the collection bottle from time to time.

For those who prefer more privacy to pump, lots of shopping centres offer baby care rooms which are quiet spaces that can be used for expressing as well as for nursing. They are also a more hygienic option than pumping in the toilets.

If you have a car, it can provide another space in which to pump a bit more privately. You can get car adaptors for the charger of your breast pump, although this will only work while the car engine is running. If you are a passenger, there is no reason not to pump while on route, which can be useful for longer journeys. If you are the driver though the law is a little less clear – under the Australian Road Rules 2008, Rule 297, a driver cannot drive unless they have complete control of the car. Arguably it is fine to pump with a hands-free pump or bra while driving, as long as you have full control of the car. Make sure you are stationary before hooking up or unhooking your pump and don't drive while pumping unless you are completely confident that you can do so safely and without needing to take your hands off the wheel.

Make sure you have your pump fully charged before you set out and that you have all the parts and bottles you need. If you are going to be out for more than one session, plan how to wash and sterilise your pump, or take enough spare parts to cover all the sessions. Think too about how you will store and transport the milk – freshly expressed milk can sit out at room temperature for up to 4 hours, but if you'll be out longer and won't be feeding the milk to your baby within that time, you might need to take a cool bag or make use of a fridge if one is available. If you have your baby with you, the best thing is to use the expressed milk for your baby's feed while you are out.

## What to do with your baby while you pump

Dedicating two hours plus of your day to pumping is already a big ask but when you factor in that you also need to care for a baby during this time, it can all feel a bit mind-boggling, especially at the start. Babies come with a wide range of different temperaments and have a varying degree of tolerance for amusing themselves. Even if you are lucky enough to get one of those mythical babies who will regularly lie happily cooing to themselves for long stretches of time, you are bound to have the occasional bad day. If you are exclusively pumping, this can be challenging as the demands of pumping don't necessarily gel well with your baby's insistence that you never sit still for longer than five minutes. A hands-free bra and a pump with a good degree of portability can help to a certain extent, as you'll at least not be completely tethered to one spot. Here are some other options to try:

## Put someone else on baby care

If someone else is around - whether that is your partner, a family member, or a friend – let them be in charge of the baby while you are on pumping duty.

## Have them on your lap

In some ways, newborns can be easier in this regard, as most do sleep a lot of the day (just not necessarily at the times you would like them to). If your baby likes to be held while they sleep, you can simply give them a cuddle while you pump, although you might still want a cosy place to lay them down close by for when your pumping session ends and you want to unhook. Even when wakeful, many newborns prefer to be in your arms than put down and are more likely to give you some peace to pump if you have them on your lap. A lot of babies prefer to be walked or danced than to sit still with you so a rocking chair or one of those big bouncy exercise balls can help give them the motion they desire while still allowing you to sit down.

## Feed them while you pump

If you have gone for a pumping routine that involves pumping when your baby feeds, you can occupy your baby by giving them a bottle while you pump. Get everything ready before you sit down and hook up your pump first before starting your baby on their feed. Just be careful of not knocking your pump when it is time to burp your baby – try laying them over one arm or your leg rather than your shoulder. If it is all feeling a little crowded on your lap, a nursing pillow can be useful to prop your baby on while giving them their bottle.

## Play with them

With younger babies, this might just look like holding them on your lap, singing songs, and playing peekaboo. With older babies, you might need to sit on the floor (make sure you have something to lean against to prevent a sore back) so that you can play more freely. Depending on your coordination while pumping, you could use the time for some baby massage, which is a soothing activity for you both.

## Use a bouncy chair or jungle gym

Bouncy chairs are a useful and usually inexpensive bit of baby kit. Many babies seem to be happier propped up in one in the early weeks than they are lying down. Once they are beginning to grab for things it can be trickier to have the baby on your lap while pumping, as they will otherwise be making a determined bid for your pump, hair, or anything else that comes into reach. Many bouncy chairs come with dangly toys they can practice their grabbing on instead. For slightly older babies who are not yet pulling up to stand, a baby jungle gym can keep your baby entertained with lots of colours, textures, and toys for them to grab.

## Pump while they nap

As your baby gets older, they will likely fall into a more consistent nap routine, which means you can more reliably use their sleep time for your pumping sessions. Many babies go through a short napping stage where they will only sleep for 45 minutes at a time – if your baby is doing this, make sure you sit down to pump as soon as they are asleep so you don't get interrupted. There will inevitably be the odd day where they are refusing to go down at all, but it is generally easier to pump during naptime with older babies, especially once they are mobile and getting into everything.

## Set up a yes space

If your baby is mobile and pumping while they nap doesn't always work out, you can set up a yes space – this could be a whole room or a smaller area of a larger room. The idea is to create a space that is as free as possible of hazards and full of interesting, baby-appropriate toys and materials to explore. This gives your baby somewhere they can play and move safely while you pump so that you aren't constantly having to direct them away from things they shouldn't touch. Depending on your baby's temperament, you can either set up your pumping station in the same room or somewhere within earshot. Some babies seem to become more absorbed with their play when they can't see you, others will prefer to know you are close by.

## When nothing else works

Sometimes there is nothing you can do to keep your baby happy for the 15 or so minutes it takes you to pump. You might be able to delay pumping a little if it is just the one fussy patch in an otherwise smooth day, but if you are desperately needing to express and can't get your baby to settle, it is OK to take the time to pump anyway. Make sure your baby is fed and has a clean nappy before you start. If you can, keep them with you so you can continue to comfort them with your presence, but if it is all feeling too much, putting them down somewhere safe just for a short time is fine too. It feels horrible when your baby is crying and you can't help them – taking some time to make sure you are comfortable and have expressed the milk you need means you can go back to them without feeling distracted and stressed by the need to pump. This will give you a better chance of being able to stay calm while you care for them.

## Pumping when you have older children

As if balancing the needs of a new-born and regular pumping sessions weren't enough, having older children to care for too can really add to the load, especially if they are toddlers or preschoolers who need a lot of your time. Your older children might also be struggling to adjust to having a new sibling and might be anxious for your attention. It helps to have a plan in advance on how to keep your older children occupied while you are pumping.

## Special toys

You could put together an activity box or some special toys that your older children only play with while you are pumping. Before you sit down to pump, get their box out so they have something to keep themselves occupied. Rotate these occasionally so that they don't lose their charm. For slightly older children, puzzle or sticker books are good to keep them occupied.

## Read stories

A good sedentary activity that can also be a sweet bonding moment with your older children is to have them snuggle up with you and a book during your pumping session. If you have school-age children, perhaps they could even read to you instead of you reading to them. As with toys, it is a good idea to have a few special books set aside for this purpose and to rotate them regularly to avoid boredom.

## Sibling playtime

If you have more than one older child, enlist the help of older siblings in entertaining the little ones. Most older children like the feeling that their parents trust them to be responsible. You might want to have some suggestions for activities planned out to avoid squabbling over what game to play.

## Arts and crafts

Sticking, painting, colouring and messy play are all good activities to absorb older children during a pump session – just make sure that whatever you offer is something they can manage without too much help from you. The downside of course is that there's generally quite a bit of mess to clear up afterwards.

## Bath-time

If your older children are water lovers, you could time one of your pumping sessions for their bath-time, or occasionally even get them to have an extra special bath in the middle of the day. Encourage them to enjoy it longer with bubbles and bath-toys. You'll need a battery-powered pump for this since most bathrooms don't have power outlets.

## Screen-time

Even if you have strict rules about screen use in your home, this season of life is one where taking advantage of the distraction power of the TV or computer makes a lot of sense. Your older children can snuggle up with you and watch their favourite show while you express.

## Get them involved

Toddlers especially like to be 'helpful' and can rarely resist the temptation to get involved with whatever you are trying to do. Redirect this helpful instinct by giving them a task to do – they could be in charge of turning your pump on for you perhaps or could act as your milk spotter to let you know if your collection bottle is getting full. Older children might be able to help with assembling your pump or could be your timekeeper.

## Set them some challenges

Children who are old enough to understand and follow basic commands can make a game out of doing challenges you set them. Perhaps they could run to the kitchen and back three times, find something red, or stand on one foot for 10 seconds. All you need to do is shout out the next challenge and it gives them a chance to burn some energy while you pump.

# QUICK TIPS FROM CHAPTER 5

## First 4-6 weeks

• pump in a way that mimics a newborn's natural feeding pattern: every 2-3 hours, including once or twice at night

• aim for a minimum of 2 hours pumping a day across 8-12 sessions

• choose to go by the clock, pump when your baby feeds, or a combination of the two

• newborns usually drink 2-3 ounces per feed

• between 1 and 6 months old, babies drink on average 25 ounces per 24 hour period

• use an app to track your pumping sessions, output, and how much your baby eats

## Middle of the night pumping

• Middle of the night sessions are important for establishing a good supply

• Aim to pump at least once at night for the first 12 weeks

• Prepare in advance

• Let your baby wake you rather than setting an alarm

• Get your partner to do the night feeds or feed and pump simultaneously

• Get a white noise machine

• Buy some angled breast shields

## Dropping night pumping sessions

- Choose your approach depending on how prone you are to blocked ducts

- You can opt to drop one session all at once

- Or gradually reduce the time or volume you pump

- Or push a session later and later until it is close enough to the next session to drop

- Use cabbage leaves or take a lecithin supplement to help with clogged duct issues

- Keep an eye on your supply

## Adapting as your baby gets older

- Expect to pump for the same amount of time but across fewer feeds

- Add the time from your dropped pumping session to the remaining sessions

- Many babies will eat roughly every 4 hours by around 3-4 months

- Keep an extra session if you want to build a freezer stash

- Use the advice from dropping night pumping if you are dropping daytime pumping sessions

## Pumping once your baby starts solids

- Start to introduce solids from around 6 months

- Keep pumping sessions the same at first

- By 10-12 months, most babies eat three meals a day

- They start to need less milk, so you can begin to drop pumping sessions without adding the extra time to other sessions

## Out and about

- Expressing breastmilk is covered by the same anti-discrimination laws as breastfeeding

- A hands-free pump like a Freemie is useful for pumping in public

- If you want to cover up, a nursing cover, loose top, scarf, blanket, or towel can be useful

- For more privacy, use a baby care room or pump in the car

- Pumping while driving is a grey area in the law - only do it if you are confident you can do so safely

## What to do with your baby while you pump

- Put someone else on baby care

- Have them on your lap

- Feed them while you pump

- Play with them

- Put the in a bouncy chair or on a baby jungle gym

- Pump while they nap

- Set up a yes space

- When nothing else works, make sure they are clean and fed and pump anyway

## Pumping when you have older children

- Have special toys or activity boxes on rotation

- Read stories

- Encourage siblings to play together

- Do arts and crafts

- Have bath-time

- Make use of screen-time

- Get them involved

- Set fun challenges

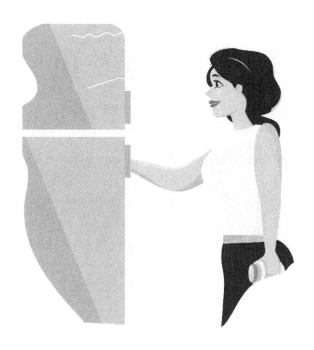

# 6. HANDLING AND STORING BREASTMILK

In the early days, you might find there isn't a big gap between expressing your breastmilk and feeding it to your baby. But as you get more established with pumping and your baby starts to go longer between feeds, you will likely be getting a bit ahead of your baby's needs, or even starting to build a freezer stash. Correctly handling and storing your breastmilk is important to make sure that it stays fresh to feed to your baby. After all, you have worked hard to get it, so you want to make sure it doesn't go to waste.

Safely storing your expressed milk is not just about use-by dates either. You are going a long way to make sure that your baby gets all the amazing benefits of your breastmilk and correct storage can ensure that your baby receives all the nutrition, antioxidants, and immune-boosting properties of your milk.

### Before you start pumping

We've talked about this a bit in previous chapters, but it is worth repeating here. Before you start pumping, you want to make sure all your equipment is clean and that you have washed your hands well in hot water and soap. The more you can prevent any contamination from the very start, the longer your breastmilk will last.

Of course, there's a limit to how much you can create a sterile environment to pump in, and it isn't necessary to go overboard. Just be sensible. Many pumps come with lids that you can use to cover the breast shields of your pump if you are interrupted in the middle of a session – a fairly frequent occurrence when you have a young baby. Make sure you have these to hand so that if you need to put your pump down for a little while you don't have to leave the collection bottles open to the air. If you are going to be pouring the milk into a different bottle or into a storage container, make sure these are also clean and sterilised, ready for use. If you will use the same collection bottle you have expressed into, have the lid to hand so you can put it straight onto the collection bottle when you unhook, minimising the time it stands open to the air.

## Storing milk

Like any other food, breastmilk is better the fresher it is. The longer it is stored for, the more nutritional benefit is lost. But in the real world, it isn't always practical or desirable to feed your milk to your baby as soon as you pump it. The likelihood is that you will want to store at least a few feeds in the fridge, and you will probably also want to build up a freezer stash, so you have a back-up available. Knowing how long breastmilk stays good for at different temperatures can help you plan ahead and make sure you don't end up having to waste valuable breastmilk.

## Keeping milk at room temperature

As if breastmilk wasn't already pretty incredible for the way it meets your baby's nutritional needs, it has the added benefit of being naturally anti-bacterial. This is excellent news for when you can't immediately refrigerate your milk, as it means you can safely leave it out at room temperature (which is defined in this case as being 16-29° Celsius) for four hours. In fact, in cooler rooms, this can be extended for as long as 6-8 hours.

You'll likely see a mixture of the four and six-hour figures recommended around the web – this is partly down to possible differences in room temperature, and partly down to the difference between what is ideal and what is acceptable in terms of milk storage. So the ideal is that milk sits out for no more than four hours, but it is still good to use if it has been out for closer to 6 hours, as long as it isn't in a very warm room. This can be especially useful for pumping when out and about, or during the night when you might not have a fridge immediately to hand.

Make sure the milk remains covered while it is sitting out. You might want to wrap it in a wet towel, if one is available, to help keep the temperature down. Insulated bottle carriers can also help to protect milk from getting too warm.

If the milk has been sat out for a while and then you refrigerate it, note that it will last for less time in the fridge before it spoils. And vice versa – freshly pumped milk is good for up to 6 hours out of the fridge but if it has already been in the fridge for a day or two, you probably want to err on the side of caution and only have it out at room temperature for 4 hours or less. If you aren't sure, give the milk a good smell or dribble a little onto a spoon or the back of your hand and taste-test it. The smell and taste of spoiled milk are pretty unmistakable so you will know if it has gone off. It is unlikely to do your baby any harm even then, but they probably won't want to drink it.

## Storing milk in the fridge and freezer

If you aren't going to use expressed milk straight away and there is a fridge to hand, the best thing is to refrigerate it as soon as possible – it will stay good longer at colder temperatures. Breastmilk can last 4-5 days in the fridge. Make sure you keep it in the main part of the fridge, ideally towards the back, which is cooler than the door and less prone to temperature fluctuations from opening and closing the door.

How long your milk will last in the freezer depends on what sort of freezer you have. If it is one of those freezer drawers that sits above your fridge, the bad news is that milk can only be stored for up to 2 weeks, although that still buys you more time than the fridge alone. But in a stand-alone freezer or one that is part of a unit with your fridge but has its own door, milk can last for 3-6 months. If you have a deep freeze, you can store milk in it for 6-12 months. As with storing milk in the fridge, you want to store milk close to the back, where it is coolest. Milk does lose more nutrients in the freezer than it does in the fridge, but the advantage of being able to lay down a good stockpile is a real advantage of using the freezer. Leave some space at the top of the container to allow the milk room to expand as it freezes.

It is a good idea to store milk in the fridge or freezer in relatively small batches so that you don't end up wasting much if your baby is less hungry than you expected or the milk goes off more quickly than it should. Many people go for 2-4 ounces per container. You can add freshly expressed milk to a batch that is already in the fridge (or freezer) as long as you chill it first. Make sure to label bags or containers with the date that you pumped the milk and how much is in there, so that you have an easy reference for when you come to use it later. If you are super-organised, you can keep the stored milk in some kind of order so you always know which one to use first – always put newer milk to the back, for example, so that older milk that needs using up is towards the front.

## Using a cooler bag

If you are on the go and won't have access to a fridge, an insulated cool bag with ice packs can keep milk fresh for up to 24 hours – good news for when you are travelling. Try not to open the bag too often and make sure the milk stays in contact with the ice packs so that it remains cold enough.

## Re-warming chilled milk

While some babies are perfectly happy to drink milk straight from the fridge, many prefer the milk to be warmed before they will accept it. The key here is to not heat it up too quickly, which destroys nutrients and can cause hot spots in the milk that might burn your baby's sensitive mouth. Don't use the microwave or boiling hot water to warm milk for these reasons. You can buy dedicated bottle warmers, but honestly standing the bottle in a cup of warm water does the job just as well and doesn't require you to buy yet another bit of new kit for your baby. It also works well out and about – most cafes and restaurants will be happy to bring you a mug of warm water to use. You can also warm milk by running your hot tap and holding the bottle under the flow, turning it occasionally to warm it through evenly.

It does take a little while to warm milk this way, which is good for preserving nutrients but not so good when you have a crying hungry baby. Once your baby settles into a more predictable routine with feeds this just means planning ahead a little to have the milk warm and waiting for them. But in the hazy newborn days or in the middle of the night you may sometimes want to cheat a little by using hot water instead of just warm water, which heats the milk up faster. Just don't leave the bottle long – milk can get too hot surprisingly quickly. After a minute or two, give the milk a gentle swirl to mix it, making sure it is warmed through evenly. Squeeze a drop or two onto the back of your hand to test the temperature before feeding it to your baby. It shouldn't feel hot – you want it at no more than body temperature.

For middle of the night feeds, if you aren't using milk expressed that night, prepare bottles in advance and have them in a cool bag by the bed. Keep a mug and a thermos of hot water to hand too. Then when your baby wakes, you can use the water from the thermos to warm the prepared milk while you or your partner change the baby's nappy or give them a cuddle.

If your baby has drunk from a bottle but has not finished the feed, the recommendation is not to keep it for more than two hours.

## Thawing frozen milk

Depending on how quickly you need the frozen milk to be ready to use, you can either choose to defrost it in the fridge overnight or use the same warm water methods described above. Milk will defrost more quickly in warm water than in the fridge. You may need to change the water a couple of times if you need the milk quickly to speed up the heat exchange.

The thawed milk will keep for 24 hours in the fridge but the current advice is not to re-freeze it after it is thawed. To avoid wastage, don't defrost any more milk than you will use in a 24-hour period.

Sometimes breastmilk that has been frozen has an odd flavour, in some cases quite a strong soapy flavour. It doesn't mean the milk has gone bad – it is down to an enzyme found in breastmilk called lipase. High levels of lipase in the milk can cause the soapy taste. Your baby might drink it perfectly happily, but if you are having an issue with high lipase and your baby won't drink the thawed milk, try scalding your expressed milk before you freeze it. To do this, heat the freshly expressed milk until bubbles start to appear around the edges, but stop before it is fully boiling. Allow the milk to cool and then you can freeze it.

Another trick to try if your baby is not sure about the flavour of thawed milk is to mix it in with fresh milk – start with half of each or two-thirds fresh milk and one third thawed. As your baby gets used to the taste of the thawed milk, you can start to slowly change the proportions until there is more frozen milk than fresh in each bottle. You might eventually get them to drink just frozen milk using this method, but if the soapy flavour is very strong or your thawed milk smells rancid, use the scalding method instead.

# QUICK TIPS FROM CHAPTER 6

## Before you start pumping

• Wash your hands

• Make sure pump parts are clean and sterilised

• Have clean, sterile storage ready

• Keep lids for bottles and covers for breast shields to hand in case you are interrupted

## Storing milk

• At room temperature: 4 hours or less is optimal, 6-8 hours acceptable, depending on the temperature of the room

• In the fridge: 4 days or less is best, 5 days is acceptable

• In a freezer drawer: 2 weeks

• In a separate freezer or a freezer unit below your fridge if it has a separate door: 3-6 months

• In the deep freeze: 6-12 months

• In a cooler bag with ice packs: 24 hours

• Keep milk towards the back in the fridge or freezer

• Label containers with the date and amount

• Store milk in small batches of 2-4 ounces

• Don't completely fill containers – leave space for the milk to expand as it cools

## Re-warming chilled milk

• Try your baby on cold milk – you may not need to warm it at all

- Do not use boiling water or the microwave in case of hot spots

- Milk retains the most nutrients when reheated slowly in lukewarm water

- If you need it faster, you can use hotter water

- Check the temperature on the back of your hand before feeding to your baby

- At night, keep a thermos of hot water to hand for warming milk

- If your baby has drunk from the bottle, use the rest within 2 hours or discard it

## Thawing frozen milk

- Thaw milk slowly in the fridge, or stand it in warm water

- Thawed milk can be kept for 24 hours in the fridge

- Do not re-freeze thawed milk

- If your thawed milk tastes very soapy, try scalding it before freezing

- If the soapy taste is mild, mixing thawed milk with fresh in a feed might help your baby get used to the flavour

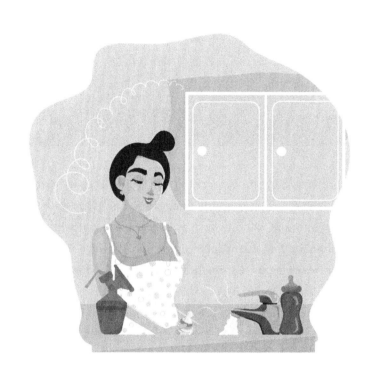

## 7. Cleaning Your Pump

Doing the washing up is never fun, but it is a necessary part of pumping. Making sure your pump is kept clean and ready to use ensures that your milk will stay fresh as long as it can and will not be exposed to bacteria that might speed up the rate at which it spoils. It also keeps it free of germs that might be bad for your baby. When you are exclusively pumping, that can mean a lot of washing up sessions, as you will need clean pump parts ready every time you pump. As discussed in earlier chapters, having spare pump parts can be a real help here in meaning you can do fewer washing sessions throughout the day and still have clean equipment when you need it.

### Which parts of the pump need to be washed?

Any part of your pump that comes into contact with your breastmilk will need to be washed after use. That means all of the collection kit, which includes:

- The breast shields

- Breast cushions (silicone inserts that line the breast shields) if your pump comes with them

- The duckbill valves that are usually found where the breast shields screw onto the collection bottles. On a Medela pump these will be small flat membrane discs instead

- The collection bottles

- The backflow protectors, usually found where the breast shields connect to the pump's tubes

You shouldn't normally need to wash the tubes that connect the pump to the breast shields in a closed system pump and definitely don't immerse the pump motor itself in water! If you do notice any condensation in the pump tubes, running the pump for a few minutes without the breast shields attached will normally sort out the problem. If you do decide to give the tubes a wash, make sure they are fully dry before you begin pumping. Again, running the pump for a few minutes with the tubes detached from the breast shields can help to clear any last drops of water.

The pump itself doesn't go anywhere near your breastmilk if it is a closed system but like anything, especially in a house with small children, it will get mucky over time. It is a good idea to wipe it down occasionally with a damp cloth or antibacterial wipe to keep it clean. If you have a rental pump or are sharing with someone else this is more important and should be done before every use.

## How to wash the pump parts

Once you are finished pumping and have safely stored your breastmilk (see previous chapter), take your pump collection kit fully apart. That means removing the valves or membranes, taking any breast cushions out of the breast shields, and taking apart the backflow protectors. Check the instructions from the manufacturer of your specific model for instructions on how to break the collection kit down into its separate parts. If you bought your pump second-hand and don't have a manual, you can usually find instructions online.

It is really important to take the collection kit apart before cleaning it because small amounts of milk can get in between the different parts and will cause mould growth if they are not fully dismantled and washed separately. This often catches people who are new to pumping out, but you will soon get used to taking your pump apart and reassembling it before use.

Even if you will not be giving the kit a full wash straight away, give it a rinse in cold running water once you finish pumping. This helps to remove milk residue and makes it easier to clean.

When you come to wash the kit properly, use a dedicated washing up tub and brush. This prevents cross-contamination from the rest of the family's dishes. Your baby's bottles can go into the same wash, of course. If you are low on storage space or will be needing to wash your pump parts away from home on a regular basis, a collapsible washing tub is a good option.

Fill the tub with hot water and dish soap. You don't need a special soap for this, your regular dishwashing soap will do fine. Wash each part of the pump thoroughly, using the dedicated brush. If you have a Medela pump, the small membranes can be easy to lose track of in the soapy water, so you might want to keep them on the side and only add them to the water at the point you are washing them. Rinse each piece of the pump under running water to remove any remaining soap.

**Note:** don't leave your breast pump parts to soak in hot water and soap for a long time – this doesn't help to make them any cleaner and can allow them to become contaminated with germs. If you are struggling to clean some areas, a 50/50 mixture of vinegar and water can help to shift stubborn milk.

The collection kit from most brands can also be put in the dishwasher but check the instructions from the manufacturer to make sure. Small pieces, such as valves and membranes, may get dislodged or

lost so it is best to place these into a small mesh bag or basket –
something that is open enough to allow the water in to wash the pieces,
but closed enough to prevent them from being lost. Use the top rack of
your dishwasher and make sure all parts are positioned so that the water
can drain out from them as the dishwasher runs through its cycle.

If your dishwasher programme includes a heated drying cycle, you
might want to use this to cut down on drying time and to sanitise your
kit.

## Drying pump parts

Once your collection kit has been washed and rinsed, you want to
let it air-dry. Don't use a towel to dry it – this can lead to germs being
transferred onto the clean pump parts from the towel. If you are in a
hurry, you can use a disposable towel. Some people even report having
used a hair-dryer or an electric hand-dryer to speed up the process.

Pump parts can take up a surprising amount of space, especially if
you are washing several sets at a time and bottles too. If you have room,
try to find somewhere apart from your general washing and cooking
area to lay your kit out to dry to prevent cross-contamination. Make
sure you have a clean surface to put the parts on – you want to use a
drying rack to raise the pieces up slightly so they can dry. If you are
short on room, a tiered drying rack can help by using vertical space
instead of counter space.

## Sterilising pump parts

Since most homes aren't sterile environments, technically what
you are doing to your pumping kit and your baby's bottles is sanitising
them rather than sterilising, but most of us think of this process as
sterilising, so that is how we will refer to it here too. If your baby is less
than three months old, was premature, or has a compromised immune
system, sterilising your equipment is especially important to reduce the
chance of passing on germs to your baby and you should be doing it at

least once a day. If your baby is older and healthy, then you can do it less often.

Sterilising uses either heat or chemicals to further kill off germs that might have survived the washing process. There are three main options:

## Cold water sterilising

This involves fully immersing all the parts of your collection kit in a sterilising solution. These solutions either come ready made up or as tablets which are then dissolved into cold water. Everything should be full submerged in the liquid. Cover the container with an airtight lid to keep the kit under the liquid. Leave the equipment in the solution for as long as specified by the manufacturer – usually around 15 minutes. The liquid needs to be changed every 24 hours if you are using it for more than one batch of equipment.

When you remove the pump parts from the liquid, rinse them with cooled boiled water and allow them to air-dry before use. You can leave the parts in the liquid until you are ready to use them again, which keeps them sanitised for longer. Keep the lid in place until you want to remove the parts.

This method does mean you have to keep buying the sterilising solution or tablets, which can add up. You may also be concerned about soaking your pump and baby's bottles in the solution but as long as you go for a brand that is marked as safe to use for baby-feeding equipment, there is no need to worry. Cold water sterilisation can be especially useful if you are away travelling without an easy way to boil or steam your pumping equipment, or if the manufacturer of your pump recommends against using boiling or steaming.

## Steaming

Dedicated steamers for sterilising baby equipment can be found in most chemists or baby shops. Sometimes you can even get a package deal with your baby's bottles. There are two main types – stand-alone electric steamers, or ones that go into the microwave. Check the user manual for your pump before using a steam steriliser, as some parts may not be able to be sterilised this way.

Follow the instructions on the steamer – generally they work pretty quickly, needing just 10 minutes or less to sterilise your equipment. Let the steriliser cool down before you remove your pump kit, especially if you have a microwave steamer, as it may be extremely hot. You can leave the parts in the steamer until you are ready to use them again. Just keep the lid in place.

Steam sterilising is quick and efficient and there is no need to rinse equipment after using this method. It does require a specific bit of kit, however, which you may not want to lug with you if you are travelling.

## Boiling

You don't need any special equipment or solutions for this method, just a large pan with a close-fitting lid and a heat source. If you can, try to use the pan only for sterilising and not for cooking, which can lead to cross-contamination. Check first that all the parts of your collection kit are suitable for boiling.

Make sure that the parts are fully submerged under the water and use the lid to keep them beneath the surface of the liquid. Boil the water for five minutes, then turn off the heat. Leave the pan until it has fully cooled down before trying to remove the pump parts or you risk burns from the hot water. Again, you can leave the equipment in the covered pan until you are ready to use them again, although you need to allow for drying time too.

This is a low cost method as it doesn't require you to purchase extra equipment – even if you don't already have a pan large enough, you can use one you buy for cooking when your baby is done with breastmilk. But it can cause your pump parts to need replacing more quickly. Be careful not to leave the water boiling for longer than 5 minutes and check pump parts after each sterilisation to make sure there is no damage.

# QUICK TIPS FROM CHAPTER 7

## Washing

• Wash any part of your pump that has come into contact with breastmilk

• Tubes and the pump motor don't need washing

• Take the collection kit apart to wash

• Rinse equipment in cold running water as soon as you are done pumping

• Use a dedicated washing tub and brush

• Wash by hand in hot soapy water and then rinse clean, or use the top rack of your dishwasher

## Drying

• Don't use a towel to dry pump parts

• Air-drying is best

• You can also use a disposable paper towel

## Sterilising

• For young or immune-compromised babies, sterilise equipment at least once a day

• For older, healthy babies you can sterilise less regularly

• Options are: cold water sterilisation, steaming, and boiling

• Make sure pump parts are suitable for the method you select

• Allow equipment to cool before removing from the steriliser

- Keep parts in the steriliser, with the lid on, until you are ready to use them again

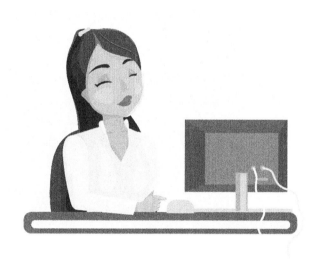

## 8. PUMPING AT WORK

Although not everyone returns to work after having a baby, many of us do, which brings all the challenges of balancing working life and parenthood. If your baby is still drinking breastmilk when you return to work then you have a choice to make – either to continue to pump while you are at work, or to wean your baby onto formula (or perhaps cows' milk if they are over one year old).

If you are already exclusively pumping at the point your return to work beckons, the good news is that you are ahead of the game. You are already familiar with using your pump, probably have a regular pumping routine worked out, and hopefully have all the equipment you need to pump comfortably away from home. There are a few extra things to think about, such as storing and transporting breastmilk, and how to find the space and time to pump at work, but the past few months of pumping have put you in a good place to successfully continue to express milk while at work.

### Know your rights

Under the Federal Sex Discrimination Act 1984, it is illegal to discriminate against breastfeeding mothers. State legislation backs this up, although the exact wording varies from state to state. What this means for you is that if you wish to pump at work, your employer must make reasonable accommodation to allow you to do so. This should include finding you a clean, private place to pump (which is not a toilet) and allowing you to organise your breaks to fit your pumping schedule.

Of course, there is a big range in what might be considered 'reasonable' and the application of this legislation will vary from workplace to workplace. If your employer is signed up to the Australian Breastfeeding Association's Breastfeeding Friendly Workplaces scheme, they should already be well set-up to allow you to pump at work – part of the criteria for the scheme is that there is a suitable space available for pumping and that the employer will allow you the time and support you need while you are still expressing milk for your baby.

Larger organisations are more likely to be arranged in a way that allows you to pump at work easily – as a general rule, they have more space, may have had people pumping at work in the past, and have a formal HR team and policies to cover support for newly returned parents. If your employer is a smaller organisation you may need to do a bit more of the groundwork, especially if you are the first person they have had needing to pump at work. Space might also be more of an issue in a smaller building.

### Talking to your employer about pumping at work

The best thing is to start talking to your employer about your plans well before you actually return to work. Explain to them that you need to pump at work to provide breastmilk for your child and that you will require space and time to do this.

If you can, suggest ways that your employer might be able to accommodate you and how you will organise your working day and still give yourself time to pump. If there is a policy already in place, make sure that you know what it says so that you can point to it if necessary.

Most employers will be accommodating, especially if you can show that you have thought about the logistics and have a plan in place to make it work.

If you do hit issues with a non-sympathetic employer, you could start by asking them to read the free information available from local branches of the Australian Breastfeeding Association and on their Breastfeeding Friendly Workplaces website: https://www.breastfeeding.asn.au/workplace. Request a meeting with your HR team, if there is one, or your line manager if not, to discuss their objections. Stay firm – you have the right to request this accommodation and there is no need to be apologetic. Use this conversation to gently point them towards the state and federal legislation that covers your right to pump at work – when they realise that refusing to make reasonable adjustments to allow you to pump is against the law, most employers will come around pretty quickly!

However, if your employer is still throwing up roadblocks in your way, you might decide to escalate the issue – your starting point will usually be your workplace's complaints or grievance process, but you can also ask for outside help via the Fair Work Ombudsman, who work with employees and workplaces to ensure fair practice, or the relevant state or territory anti-discrimination body.

Most employers will want to do the right thing, so the likelihood is that you won't encounter any serious objections. Often the hardest thing is to keep firm on your pumping goals once you are back at work and get caught up in the usual flurry of your daily tasks. Setting an alarm on your phone or blocking pumping time in your work calendar can help to remind you to keep the time free.

**Where to pump?**

Larger workplaces may have a dedicated lactation room that you can use to pump, which should be a clean space with comfortable seating, and ideally a sink you can use to rinse your pumping equipment. Many work sites don't have the space to offer a dedicated room just for pumping, but a first-aid room or prayer room is a good alternative. If neither of these are available, an unused office or meeting room might be an option instead.

With the development of discreet, hands-free pumps like the Freemie, you may not even need to go to a separate room to pump. Because these pumps have breast shields that just sit inside a regular bra, you can wear them beneath your clothes and pump without it being noticeable. If your work is mainly desk-based, using a Freemie means you can pump and work at the same time. This can be a bonus if you are struggling to arrange enough breaks to fit your pumping schedule. If your work is more physical, a Freemie might still be useful, but it won't stand up to vigorous movement, so if this is a regular part of your work, you will want to arrange your breaks accordingly.

**When to pump?**

Obviously, the ideal scenario is that you will be able to continue the same pumping schedule when you return to work. However, paid lactation breaks are not currently enforced by Australian law, which may mean you have to do some negotiating to align your breaks with your schedule.

If your workplace is accredited under the Breastfeeding Friendly Workplaces scheme, then you should be able to agree additional short, paid breaks to allow you to pump according to your desired schedule. If your employer is not accredited, but is sympathetic to your pumping requirements, they will hopefully be willing to allow you to take an extra break or two if needed without deducting it from your paid hours.

The flexibility of your work schedule will have a big role to play in how easily you can fit pumping into your working day. If you do shift work, it may be more difficult to get breaks at the time you would like than if you work a 9-5 office job. If your employer is not open to you taking additional paid breaks, explore whether you can take an unpaid break by making up the time at the end of the day. Depending on how flexible your workload is, might you be able to split a longer lunch break into two short breaks to get the time you need to pump? If you do shift work, can you agree a shift pattern with your employer that means your work fits around your pumping schedule?

You may need to compromise a little on the exact time of your pumping sessions in order to balance pumping and the demands of your working schedule. If you know in advance of returning to work what your general routine will look like, you can start to nudge your pumping schedule to match.

As with finding the space to pump, a Freemie or other hands-free pump can make fitting pumping sessions into your work schedule slightly easier, because you can use it to pump while you are working. Again, this depends on the nature of your work – it is easier to pump on the job if you are sat at a computer than if you are on the go all day.

## Storing milk at work

Hopefully, you have access to a fridge while at work – most workplaces have a lunchroom or kitchen with a fridge for employees to use. You can store breastmilk in a shared fridge without any issue, but it is a good idea to make sure it is well labelled – you don't want one of your colleagues accidentally adding it to their morning coffee. Just like at home, keep milk in the main part of the fridge, towards the back, and not in the door.

If no fridge is available in your workplace, an insulated cooler bag with ice packs can keep milk fresh for 24 hours, which should give you plenty of time to get expressed milk home to your own fridge. Again, it is a good idea to label the bag clearly so that your colleagues know it belongs to you. Depending on the length of your commute and the temperature, you may want a small cooler bag even if there is a fridge available, for transporting milk home.

## Washing your pump at work

Depending on how many times you need to pump during your working day, you may prefer just to give your collection equipment a rinse in the sink of your workplace's kitchen or lactation room and then wash it thoroughly when you get home. Taking enough spare pump parts to last for the full day means you can still do this even when you are expressing multiple times during your working day.

Lugging a pump and spare equipment, plus your expressed milk, plus whatever else you need for your day at work, can be a pain though, especially if you commute on public transport, or there is no parking near your workplace. If you have the funds and a secure place to leave it, you might consider having a second pump that lives at your workplace, instead of taking it back and forth every day.

You could just keep the pump motor and tubes at work and transport the collection equipment so that you can clean it at home or, if your workplace has the space for you to wash and dry your equipment on site, you could keep everything you need there to avoid carrying it. Make sure you use a dedicated washing up tub and brush to clean your pumping equipment at work to avoid contamination with the rest of your colleagues' washing up. The bonus of keeping everything at work is that you are less likely to forget an important part of your pump and be stuck unable to express milk without it.

## Breastmilk and childcare

Just as anti-discrimination laws protect your right to pump at work, they protect your right to ask whoever cares for your child to feed them with your expressed milk. Depending on the type of childcare you choose for your baby, their caregiver may or may not already be familiar with the safe storage of breastmilk and how to warm it up for your baby. You can always leave them with some instructions at first until they get used to handling it. The Australian Breastfeeding Association have a free leaflet available too which is a useful resource to pass to your child's carer.

It can be helpful to take the milk for your baby already prepared in bottles, so that it is easy for their carers to prepare their feeds. Make sure bottles are well labelled with your baby's name and the time they should be given the feed, especially if they are likely to drink different amounts at different times of day. You can take milk in a cooler bag and your childcare provider should have a fridge available to store it in during the day. With any luck, they might wash the bottles for you too but if that isn't part of the service, ask them to give the bottles a rinse under cold water to remove the milk residue so that you can wash them more thoroughly at home.

## Know your rights

• Anti-discrimination legislation protects your right to pump at work

• Your employer must make reasonable adjustments to allow you to pump

• Some employers are accredited as Breastfeeding Friendly Workplaces

## Talking to your employer

• Talk to your employer about your plans to pump before you return to work

• Suggest ways to make pumping work logistically

• Know your workplace's policy if there is one

• If your employer is unsympathetic, make sure they understand that refusal to make reasonable accommodation is against the law

• If you experience discrimination as a result of requesting accommodations to allow you to pump at work, you can contact the Fair Work Ombudsman for help

## Where to pump?

• Your employer should make a clean, private space available for you to pump

• This could be a lactation room, first aid room, prayer room, or other unused space

• A Freemie pump, or similar, can allow you to pump while working

## When to pump?

- Paid lactation breaks are not currently enforced by Australian law

- Some workplaces will allow you to take extra paid breaks anyway

- You could also take unpaid breaks and make the time up at the end of the day, or use your existing breaks more flexibly

- If you do shift work, negotiate with having your shifts fit around your pumping

**Storing milk**

- Milk can be stored in a shared fridge

- If no fridge is available, use an insulated cooler bag

- Make sure all expressed milk is well labelled

**Washing your pump equipment**

- Rinse collection equipment and then wash thoroughly at home

- Take enough spare pump parts to last the whole day

- Having a second pump can save on carrying

- If washing at work, use a dedicated wash tub and brush

**Breastmilk and childcare**

- Your childcare provider must accommodate you by feeding your expressed milk to your child

- Leave instructions on safe breastmilk handling

- Label bottles well

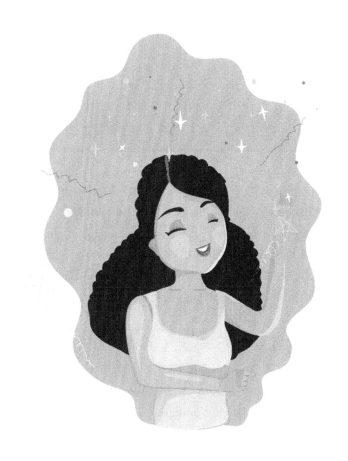

# 9. MENTAL HEALTH

Being a new parent is an absolute emotional rollercoaster. Even if this isn't your first child, your life has just changed radically. On top of that, you are sleep-deprived, hormonal, and recovering from giving birth. If you have had a complicated delivery, or your baby is premature or unwell, there's medical stress thrown into the mix. And in the later months, there is the constant juggling of everyone's needs, often coupled with loneliness and isolation.

Every parenting journey has its ups and downs, but there are some pressures that are specific to pumping families. When so much advice is focused on nursing, it can sometimes feel like you are the only one in the world taking the exclusive pumping route. There are groups and consultants focused on helping nursing mothers, but far fewer support mechanisms in place for those who are pumping.

That's not to say at all that exclusively pumping only comes with emotional lows. The pride and satisfaction in knowing you have overcome obstacles to successfully feed breastmilk to your baby is empowering. The community around exclusive pumpers might be smaller, but it is a very supportive one. When pumping is going well, you can feel like a rock-star. If things are fine, that's awesome news –

feel free to skip this chapter for now and come back later if you need to. But for those times when you aren't feeling so great, this chapter covers some of the common emotions that come up for exclusive pumpers and gives some suggestions for how you can deal with them.

Please note: The advice in this chapter is only a starting point and should not be used in place of medical advice. If you are struggling with your mental health (at any time, not just as a new parent) reaching out for professional help can make a world of difference. You do not have to suffer on your own. Prioritising your mental wellness is part of being a good parent. Speak to your doctor, find a therapist, or reach out to a mental health charity. In particular, PANDA specialise in supporting people struggling with perinatal anxiety and depression. They have online resources and a free helpline. Call 1300 726 306, 9am – 7.30pm Mon – Sat(AEST/AEDT) or email support@panda.org.au for email support during helpline hours.

## Grief

For a lot of exclusively pumping parents, grief and disappointment top the list of emotions that are thrown up by this journey. Chances are, you were making plans for how you would care for your baby well before they were actually born. When the reality is different from what you pictured, it can be difficult to cope with. If you wanted to nurse, you might struggle to come to terms with the different turn your road has taken. Grief can be a strange thing too – you might not feel it at the point you decide to exclusively pump, only to have it smack you in the face further down the line.

If you are dealing with grief at not being able to nurse your child, the first step is to acknowledge the feeling. Name it. Don't try to push it away or to prevent yourself from feeling it. Gently remind yourself that exclusively pumping to feed your baby is an amazing thing to do but try to be patient with yourself if it takes time to work through the feelings.

Talking to someone can be really helpful – if you have a friend or family member who you can trust to listen and hold space for you, rather than trying to 'fix' the issue, share your feelings with them. If there is no one already in your life who can do this for you, reach out to other exclusively pumping parents, either in real-life or online. They are likely to have experienced similar emotions. You could also consider speaking to a counsellor or therapist. Make sure you have time each day with your baby where you aren't pumping or feeding them or otherwise caretaking – time that is just about fun and bonding, not your feeding journey.

**Guilt**

There is a lot of pressure to breastfeed your baby – and for most people, when they say breastfeed, what they actually mean is nurse. Even if you planned to pump before your baby was born, the constant barrage of messages about how you should be feeding your baby can still have an effect. Some parents feel guilty that they have given up on nursing or wonder if they have taken the easy route out.

Firstly, to reassure you – you have not taken the easy way out and however you choose to feed your baby is absolutely fine. Guilt, sadly, is part of being a parent, especially in the age of social media which can quickly have you believing that other parents are doing everything better. It is OK to put up some boundaries to protect your mental health – indeed it is healthy. If your mothers' group is full of nursing chat, or that social media account waxes lyrical about the 'special' bond of nursing, consider whether you need them in your life. Find people, in real life and online, who make you feel supported, seen, and encouraged.

You might want to write yourself a letter for times when you are doubting yourself. Remind yourself of the reasons why exclusively pumping is the right choice for you and your family, that you are doing a fantastic job feeding breastmilk to your baby, and pumping *is* breastfeeding. It is just not nursing, and that is OK. Read the letter back whenever you need a pep talk and don't have someone else around to cheerlead for you.

**Frustration**

Here's the thing about pumping – it's not fun. In fact, it is often boring, annoying, and inconvenient. And then you have to do the washing up. So it is no surprise if you sometimes find yourself feeling frustrated or overwhelmed at the thought of yet another pumping session.

Start by making your pumping as comfortable and hassle-free as you can. There's nothing that can make it your favourite activity, but the tips in the earlier chapters of this book should help to make it less of a chore.

Try to get out of the house regularly. A change of scene and some fresh air can do wonders for your mental state. If you can, make space for some time without your baby – this can be easier said than done, especially in the early days. But an adults-only trip out, even if it is just for a quick coffee, can help you to feel more like a human being and less like a milk machine. If a baby-free trip out isn't possible right when you need it, perhaps a shorter self-care break is an option instead – a long bath, half-an-hour to read a book, or a power nap. Sleep deprivation is an unavoidable part of having a young baby but can make everything feel a hundred times harder. So if the opportunity arises to get some sleep, take it.

Humour can also go a long way to help diffuse tension – online exclusive pumping communities are full of jokes, memes and gifs that offer the relief of knowing you aren't the only one going through the ups and downs of pumping. On the other hand, sometimes what you really need is a good rant to get the way you feel off your chest. As with dealing with guilt, surround yourself with people who will buoy you up and encourage you when you are disheartened. Ideally people who won't mind if you sometimes need to unleash on them.

When the frustration gets too much and you start to consider throwing in the towel, give yourself a short-term goal to work towards. Months, or even weeks, might be too overwhelming at this point. You could tell yourself that you will get to the end of the week, or the end of the day, or even to the end of your next pumping session. When you get there, make another short-term goal.

After you have reached a few short-term goals, you can start to make longer term plans, if the frustration begins to fade. If it doesn't, you might want to look at making some changes: Do you need to reassign household tasks so that your partner is doing more? Can someone take the baby for an hour or two on a regular basis so you can go out or catch up on some sleep? Are funds available for a cleaner or other help? Do you want to consider supplementing with formula? Or is it time to think about weaning? Notice how those options make you feel when you read them – if your heart rises or sinks at one or other of them, that can tell you which ones are right for you at this time.

### Anxiety

Being a new parent can be an anxious time – there's so much to learn and babies throw all sorts of curveballs at us. There is always something new to worry about. Along with the usual concerns that come with a new baby, pumping brings a host of issues of its own, especially if your journey has been less than smooth. Lots of pumping mothers worry about their supply, bonding with their baby when they are having to spend so much time pumping, and what will happen if they have to miss a pumping session. While worrying occasionally is part of being a parent, if your worry about pumping has spilled over into anxiety and is making you feel stressed, it is time to take some action.

Try to separate out the reality from the anxiety – which parts of your worries are rooted in truth? For example, if you are constantly anxious about your supply, look at how much you are pumping daily and how much your baby drinks daily. Write down the figures so you can see whether your concern is based on facts or on the stress of being a new, sleep-deprived parent. You might find that it is your mental state which is causing the issue, not the facts. In this case, concentrating on what *is* rather than what might be is a useful technique for disrupting anxious thoughts. When you notice your anxiety rising, take some deep breaths (there are apps available on your phone which can help with this) and remind yourself of the truth of the situation.

If your worries do have some basis in truth, making a game plan for how you will address the issue can make you feel more in control. Use the tips from this book, speak to a lactation consultant, or crowdsource ideas from an online exclusive pumping community. Write down your plan and discuss it with your partner. When you feel anxious thoughts come up, revisit your plan to reassure yourself you have it under control. Try to give yourself some grace to make changes that you need to without judgement. If supplementing with formula is what you need to do to get peace of mind, for example, supplement with formula. Your baby needs you far more than they need a breastmilk-only diet.

Talking through how you are feeling and asking for support is always a good idea when you are struggling with anxious thoughts. A friend or family member might be able to help you challenge the narrative that is causing your worries and reframe your thoughts in a more positive way. Therapy can also be helpful for all kinds of anxiety – many therapists focus in this area and you might be able to find someone with a particular specialty in parenting.

## Sudden sadness or anxiety that comes when you pump

Not all the feelings associated with pumping are psychological. Some people suffer with a condition called D-MER, which is short for Dysphoric Milk Ejection Reflex. If your letdown is accompanied by a feeling of sadness, anxiety, or depression that comes on suddenly and stops once your first letdown is over or you stop pumping, you might be experiencing D-MER. It is caused by a drop in dopamine, the feel-good hormone which plays a role in feelings of pleasure and reward. There are varying degrees of severity, from a mild feeling of sadness to an overwhelming feeling of depression. Because D-MER is physiological, it is as much of a reflex as jerking your leg when someone hits your knee. You can't stop it from happening, but that doesn't mean you need to suffer alone.

Sometimes, just knowing what is happening is enough to make D-MER manageable – it won't stop the feelings, but it can give you the reassurance of understanding why the sadness arises and that it will pass. You might also want to track the feelings, to see if there are any links with other things going on in your life, such as diet, stress, caffeine consumption, or the amount of sleep you are getting.

In many cases, D-MER improves and gradually disappears as your baby gets older. But if your symptoms are severe, you might want to speak to your doctor about getting further help. Although there is not yet an approved medical treatment for D-MER, antidepressants that raise your dopamine levels may help. Speak to your doctor about finding one that is safe to take while you are pumping.

## Postpartum depression

It is normal to go through a whole gamut of emotions when parenting a young baby – sometimes you find yourself swinging from blissed out to completely overwhelmed and back all in the space of five minutes. Most new mothers find they go through a very emotional stage in the first week or two of giving birth – caused by the changing hormones of labour and birth, this is often termed 'the baby blues' and usually passes within a month.

For many new parents though, the baby blues don't shift but continue or worsen, becoming postpartum depression. Postpartum depression can also appear later on. Key signs include increased levels of irritability, difficulty in falling asleep even though you are exhausted, and increased levels of anxiety. If you think you might have postpartum depression, it is important to reach out for help – both from your friends and family and from healthcare professionals. Again, PANDA's free helpline is a good first port of call.

There hasn't been any research specifically into the frequency of postpartum depression in the exclusively pumping community. However, some studies have found a link between difficulties in nursing in the early weeks and developing postnatal depression later on. Marshalling your support system from the start and making your mental health a priority, including giving yourself some time for self-care, are good ways to ensure you will notice if you are experiencing the symptoms of postpartum depression.

# QUICK TIPS FROM CHAPTER 9

## Grief

• Common among exclusive pumping families when there was a strong desire to breastfeed before the baby was born

• Acknowledge the feeling and allow yourself to time to work through it

• Speak to a sympathetic friend or family member, or reach out to other exclusively pumping parents

• Consider therapy

## Guilt

• Can be caused by a focus on nursing as the 'best' way to feed your baby

• Remember: pumping is breastfeeding. You are doing an amazing thing for your baby

• Keep strong barriers: prioritise spending time with people who help and support you

• Write a letter to remind yourself why exclusive pumping is the best option for your family

## Frustration

• Pumping can cause you to feel frustrated and overwhelmed

• Make pumping as comfortable and hassle-free as you can

• Get out of the house regularly, without the baby on occasion

• Make time for self-care

• Find a community to support you with humour and space to rant

- Make short-term goals

- Make changes to lighten the load

**Anxiety**

- Some people experience anxiety around pumping and supply

- Use deep breathing to help calm yourself – apps are available to help

- Focus on the truth of the situation

- If issues are present, make a game plan to give yourself control

- Reach out for support from friends and family

- Consider therapy

**Sudden sadness and anxiety associated with pumping**

- May be symptomatic of Dysphoric Milk Ejection Reflex (D-MER)

- A physiological reaction, not a psychological one

- Read more into D-MER to understand what you are feeling

- Keep track of symptoms and anything that lessens or worsens them

- In many cases, D-MER will disappear as your baby ages

- If your symptoms are severe, speak to your doctor about medication

**Postpartum depression**

- 'The baby blues' are common in the first month after birth

- For some, they will not ease but become postpartum depression

- Look out for irritability, insomnia and anxiety

- Reach out for help from friends, family and medical professionals

- PANDA have a free helpline: Call 1300 726 306, 9am – 7.30pm Mon – Sat(AEST/AEDT) or email support@panda.org.au for email support during helpline hours

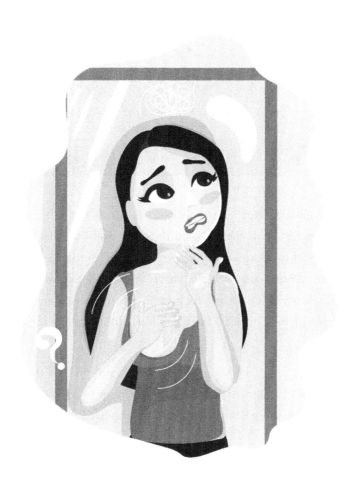

# 10. TROUBLESHOOTING: YOU

We've looked already at supply issues (chapter 4) and mental health (chapter 9). This chapter is for the other problems that can sometimes be thrown up when you are pumping; from clogged ducts and mastitis to pump issues. We'll look at the common issues that can affect you when you are exclusively pumping and discuss some ways to troubleshoot them. The next chapter will look at issues that can affect your baby.

Pumping can feel a bit strange, but it shouldn't hurt. A tingling, tugging sensation is normal, but not nipple pain or breast pain. If you are experiencing pain when you pump, then you need to make some adjustments.

## Breast shield size

It is very important that you are using the right size breast shield. If you are experiencing pain when pumping, the first thing to check is that the breast shields you are using are the right size for you. As well as pain, signs that your breast shields are not the right size include;

• Your nipple looks either very red, or white, when you pump or just after finishing pumping.

- Your nipple rubs against the side of the breast shield while pumping

- Your areola (the area around your nipple) is being pulled into the breast shield

If any of these are happening, you need a different size of breast shield. To get the sizing right, measure the diameter of your nipple. Just the nipple itself, not the areola. Use the sizing information available from your pump or breast shield manufacturer to order the right size. If the size you need isn't available from your pump's manufacturer, you can try an alternative breast shield – Pumpin' Pals are one option that offer a wide-range of different sizes.

You may need to change breast shield size at different points in your pumping journey as your breasts change according to your supply. So even if you have been using your breast shields for some time without issue, it is still worth checking that the size is right for you.

It is also a good idea to use a lubricant on your breast shields to help your nipple move smoothly in the breast shield while you pump. There are plenty of nipple creams on the market, and you could also use coconut oil. Nipple creams, coconut oil, and breastmilk are all soothing if your nipples are feeling dry and sensitive, particularly in the early days of pumping.

## Suction level

Another one to check is the suction level you are using on your pump. It can be tempting to crank up the suction in the hope that will lead to a more efficient pumping session, but the reverse is often true. Pumping at too high a suction level can cause nipple pain and can prevent good milk flow because it squeezes your breast, compressing the milk ducts just below the skin. One study found that mothers were able to express the most milk in a fifteen-minute session when they used their pumps at the strongest suction that felt comfortable, and no higher.

To find the right suction level for you, once your letdown has begun and you have your pump in expression mode, gradually increase the suction level until it feels uncomfortable. Then go back one. This is the maximum suction that you can use comfortably and should allow you to use your pump efficiently and without pain. You may find that the level you need changes from pumping session to pumping session, so make adjustments as needed each time you use your pump, rather than assuming that what worked yesterday will be right today.

**Yeast infection / thrush**

Yeast infections can be another cause of nipple or breast pain. They are most common in nursing mothers, who often find they and their baby pass the infection back and forth, but can affect pumping parents too. Thrush can be caused by an imbalance in good bacteria, often as the result of taking antibiotics, or a lowered immune system. You might experience a burning or stabbing pain in your nipple or in the breast itself. Your nipples might become shiny, cracked, or red.

If you suspect you have thrush, go to your doctor to confirm the diagnosis. They should be able to prescribe an anti-fungal cream to treat the infection. Your baby will need to be checked too, as they might have picked up the infection from your pumped milk. Generally, you and your baby will both be treated if you are diagnosed with thrush because it is easy for the infection to be passed between you.

The difficult decision when you have been pumping with thrush is what to do with the milk, which could carry the yeast infection. You can continue to feed your baby your milk while you are both being treated, and the milk you pumped before the infection is also fine to use. But once you are both thrush-free, the milk that you pumped while you had the yeast infection could reinfect your baby. Unfortunately, freezing the milk won't kill the yeast. If you have plenty of milk, you might decide just to dump the milk (heart-breaking though that can be). If you want to keep it, you can kill the yeast by pasteurising the milk – milk donation banks usually put milk through this process to kill any pathogens before passing it on.

## Pasteurising milk

To pasteurise your milk, you need to heat it until it reaches 60 degrees Celsius. Use a large stainless-steel pot and make sure you have a thermometer so that you can keep the milk at the right temperature. You will also want to fill your sink with ice, so that you have a way to cool the milk down again.

Heat the milk slowly, stirring it occasionally so that the heat is distributed evenly and the bottom doesn't catch. Once the milk reached 60 degrees, you need to keep it at this temperature for 30 minutes – which can be a challenge! You'll likely need to lower and raise the heat occasionally to keep it at the right temperature. Carry on stirring occasionally.

Take the pot off the heat and place it in the ice to cool it down. Keep stirring it to bring the temperature down. Once the milk reaches 4 degrees, you can place it in an air-tight container and store it in the fridge or freezer. This is the same method you'd use if your frozen milk has the soapy flavour given by excess lipase.

## Preventing yeast infections

You may be able to reduce the likelihood of yeast infection. Thrush is caused by a group of fungi called candida, which feed on sugar, so eating less sugary foods might help. Breastmilk is also high in (good) sugar and thrush likes warm, wet environments, so changing your breast pads and bra regularly is a good idea. You could also encourage the good bacteria that help keep thrush at bay by taking a probiotic supplement and making sure your diet is rich in prebiotic foods, including plenty of high fibre vegetables and whole grains.

## Nipple vasospasm

Vasospasms are a very painful narrowing of a blood vessel and can occur in your nipples during, or between, pumping sessions. You might notice your nipple turning white and they are often triggered by cold temperatures. Vasospasms can be caused by other conditions, including thrush or damaged nipples, in which case they will usually stop once the underlying issue has cleared up. But they can also be associated with a condition called Raynaud's Phenomenon, which is characterised by the sudden narrowing of blood vessels in the extremities, often in response to the cold.

If you are experiencing vasospasms in both nipples, rather than just one, they last for longer than a couple of seconds, or you also get them in your fingers or toes, it is a sign that you may have Raynaud's. This condition isn't caused by pumping, anyone can have it, but it is often mistaken for thrush because of the pain that comes with it.

Since vasospasms can be triggered by low temperatures, one way of managing them is to avoid the cold, especially while pumping. Cover your nipples as soon as you are finished pumping to keep them warm, and use a source of dry heat to warm your breasts – you can buy heat pads or DIY a rice sock by filling a cloth container, such as a sock or small bag, with rice. Warm it in the microwave for 45 seconds or so and then place it over your nipples (over your clothes so it is not too hot). Massaging your nipples gently with olive oil can also help to warm them and restore blood flow.

For the pain caused by the vasospasms, ibuprofen and paracetamol are both safe to take while pumping, but you should avoid painkillers that contain aspirin, unless advised to take them by your doctor.

Caffeine, nicotine, some medications, and oral contraceptives that contain oestrogen can all trigger vasospasms, so avoid these.

Taking a magnesium supplement may help to control symptoms – although the relationship has not yet been proven, magnesium is often thought to be reduce vasospasms associated with Raynaud's by causing the blood vessels to dilate. The recommended dose is 250-300 mg, twice a day. B6 is another supplement that is often recommended for nipple vasospasms – look for it as part of a vitamin B complex that includes niacin, as this seems to be when it is most effective. You are aiming for 100 mg of B6 twice a day, so check the content in your vitamin complex and adjust your dose accordingly.

## Milk blisters

Another possible cause of nipple pain while you are exclusively pumping is a milk blister, which is when skin grows over one of your milk duct openings, causing the milk to get backed-up behind it. You'll usually see a pale or clear spot on your nipple or areola where the pain is focused. If you compress your breast to force milk down the ducts, the blocked spot will bulge outwards, which can help in identifying the issue.

Milk blisters can get better on their own, although it usually takes a few days or even weeks. To treat them more quickly, apply wet heat to your nipple before you pump. This softens the blister and helps the milk duct reopen. Make it as hot as you can bear without burning yourself. Four times a day (more if you can), do a saline soak before you apply the hot compress. To do this, dissolve 2 teaspoons of Epsom salts per cup of very hot water, then add cool water until the solution is cool enough to soak your nipple. Follow the saline soak with the hot compress, and then pump. You can also use olive oil, soaked into cotton wool, to soften the blister.

As well as helping the milk duct to reopen, the soak and hot compress can make it possible to remove the skin that is blocking the duct. Gently rub the spot with a damp washcloth or use a clean finger, or fingernail, to pull or rub the skin loose. If you can't remove it yourself using one of these options, you could ask a doctor, nurse, or other healthcare provider to use a sterilised needle to lift the skin free.

Continue to pump while you have the milk blister, after using the hot compress, in order to clear blocked milk from the duct. Use breast compressions to help the milk move down the duct. You may want to start your session with some hand expressing on that side, to encourage the milk flow before you use your pump. Regular pumping will also help to keep the duct clear once you have removed the skin. If it is painful, take a painkiller that is safe to use while expressing, such as paracetamol.

There are also some options that you can try to prevent milk blisters forming in the first place. Avoid compressing your breasts – sleep on your back or side rather than your stomach and make sure your bra fits well and is not too tight. Underwired bras are a no-no while you are pumping. Lecithin supplements, often used to prevent clogged ducts, can also help in preventing milk blisters. If you have issues with oversupply, this can make you more prone to milk blisters – use the advice in chapter 4 to tackle your oversupply.

## Clogged ducts

Where milk blisters are caused by a blockage at the opening of a milk duct, clogged ducts occur further into the duct when it isn't properly drained. They can be caused by oversupply, not pumping often enough, or your breast being compressed – by your bra, sleeping on your front, or perhaps the strap of a bag or rucksack. Not using your pump correctly may also cause clogged ducts – see the information earlier in this chapter on breast shield sizing and suction.

If you have a clogged duct, you will usually be able to feel a lump in your breast – it might be warm and red and will likely be painful to touch. It might feel less sore immediately after you pump but can cause pain during letdown. Sometimes you might notice thickened milk appearing in your pump from the blocked duct. You might also find your supply drops a little because the clogged duct is not contributing to your pumping output.

A clogged duct can become infected, causing mastitis, so you need to sort it out straight away if you develop one. To unblock the duct, you need to get the milk moving again, which means pumping. Make sure you are fully emptying your breasts at every session and consider upping the frequency of your pumping sessions until the blockage is cleared. If you are weaning, you might not want to do this as it will bring your supply back up – see the chapter on weaning for specific advice in this case.

Before you start pumping, use wet heat to help get the milk moving. You could use a hot compress – a cloth nappy works well because it stays hot and wet longer than a simple cloth – or soak your breast in hot water. If you have a manual pump, you might want to try pumping in the shower so that the warm water can encourage good milk flow. Gently massage the affected area while you warm it – in the shower, you can use a large comb, well covered in soap, and softly draw it down your breast towards the nipple to encourage the duct to unblock.

While you are pumping, use breast compressions and massage the affected area to dislodge the blockage and clear the duct. This is a good time to use a vibrating lactation massager, which may be more efficient than massaging by hand alone. Get gravity to help by learning forward while you pump. Avoid tight bras or restrictive clothing that might make the issue worse by compressing your breast tissue.

If you are prone to clogged ducts, especially when weaning or trying to lower your supply, taking a lecithin supplement can help. Aim for 3600-4800 mg lecithin per day at first. After a few weeks without issues, you can start to gradually reduce the dose.

Exclusive pumping can make you slightly more prone to clogged ducts because the pump is less efficient than a baby at draining the milk ducts. To mitigate this, adjust the angle and position of your breast shields throughout a pumping session to make sure you are emptying all the ducts. Massage and breast compressions while pumping can also prevent issues.

**Mastitis**

Mastitis is an inflammation of the breast that causes you to feel breast-pain and swelling, and flu-like symptoms such as a fever, chills, and aching joints. It can be caused by a clogged duct that isn't cleared quickly, an infection from cracked nipples, or by allergies. Symptoms often start similarly to a clogged duct, but the pain, heat and swelling are usually much more intense. You might also see red streaks appearing on your breast starting from the affected area. It usually only affects one breast at a time, but it is possible to have it in both.

Mastitis feels horrible – it always sucks getting sick but coping with sore breasts, needing to pump, and caring for a small baby, all with flu symptoms, is a real struggle. Take care of yourself – you will need to get plenty of rest, stay well-hydrated, and eat well to give your immune system the best chance of fighting off the inflammation. If possible, get someone else to take care of the house and to help with caring for your baby so you can concentrate on getting well.

If you have had symptoms for less than 24 hours, or they are not too severe, use the same treatment as for a clogged duct. That means plenty of pumping (in bed, ideally), soaking your breasts in hot water or applying a hot compress, and massage. Use safe painkillers such as paracetamol as needed to manage the pain. Most mastitis is caused by clogged ducts, so removing the blockage will help the inflammation, although it is common for your breast to continue to feel tender for a week or so afterwards.

If your symptoms don't improve after 24 hours, are sudden or severe, are in both breasts, or are accompanied by clear signs of infection – such as pus or bleeding from your nipples, dangerously high temperature, or red streaks on your breast – speak to your doctor straight away. They will likely want you to start on antibiotics to treat the infection quickly and prevent your condition worsening. Make sure you complete the full course of the antibiotics you are prescribed, even after you feel better, to ensure the infection is fully killed off. Leaving mastitis untreated can lead to abscesses developing in your breast, so it is very important to make sure you address it quickly.

If you repeatedly suffer with mastitis and clogged ducts, try to uncover and tackle the underlying cause. If you are having issues in the same place, it could be a sign that this part of your breast is being compressed – look at the fit of your bra, how you sleep, at any bags you carry regularly, and at the fit of your baby carrier, if you use one. Your diet and hydration can have an effect too – make sure you stay well-hydrated and avoid eating too much saturated fat and too much or too little salt. A diet full of fruit and vegetables can help to build a healthy immune system, making you less prone to infection. Consider supplementing with vitamin C and a probiotic in addition to support your immune system. You are also at more risk of infection if you have been stressed, unwell, or very tired. Getting enough rest when you have a small baby is a difficult ask – get someone to help if you can so that you can get some time to nap or a lie in.

As discussed earlier, taking a lecithin supplement is an effective way to reduce your likelihood of getting blocked ducts or mastitis.

Tackling oversupply issues (see chapter 4) can also help in making you less prone to issues.

## Bad back or neck

This one is a mechanical issue rather than a pumping one per se – spending so much time pumping can cause your back to hurt, especially if you are having to sit in an odd position. Look at how you are sitting – it can be tempting to hunch forward when pumping but doing this for hours every day will cause your back to hurt. Make sure you are comfortable; use cushions or pillows to prop yourself up so that you have something to lean on. Consider investing in some angled breast shields that will allow you to pump in a more reclined position. A hands-free pump or bra can help too in allowing you to have your arms free in a comfortable position. Try to vary your position too and to move around a little during a session so that you don't get too stiff being in the same spot all the time.

## Dry or cracked nipples

Especially in the early weeks, your nipples are getting used to the constant pumping and may become dry or cracked. This is especially the case if you have been attempting to nurse and having issues. There are a number of different nipple creams available that can help to soothe and moisturise your nipples. Coconut oil is also good for this and many people swear by breastmilk – its healing properties are good for more than just feeding your baby.

Make sure you eliminate common causes of nipple pain, including breast shield size, suction, and thrush. Check your positioning too – your nipple should be in the centre of the breast shield, but it is easy to get it slightly wrong, especially at night. Make sure you are changing your breast pads frequently. Being constantly damp can irritate your nipples. Letting your nipples air dry after a pumping session may help them to heal more quickly (although should be avoided if you suffer from vasospasms).

Dry or cracked nipples can make pumping painful – unfortunately, stopping isn't really an option if you want to keep your supply up. Consider using painkillers while your nipples are healing if the pain is making you dread pumping. Try applying coconut oil or nipple cream directly to the breast shields of your pump to help lubricate it and reduce irritation. Cold compresses between pumping sessions can also be soothing – again, avoid this if you have Raynaud's.

If your nipples are cracked enough to bleed a little while you are pumping, it is still fine to feed the milk to your baby – a little bit of blood won't cause them any harm, although it can turn your milk quite an alarming colour. But be careful – there is a type of bacteria called *Serratia marsescens* that can also turn your milk red. These bacteria won't cause problems in small amounts but can be harmful to your baby if they consume them in large quantities. If you know that the red colour of your pumped milk is down to blood, it is safe to use. But if you are not sure, especially if your nipples don't appear damaged, it is best to dump the milk. Proper handling and storage of breastmilk and pumping equipment (see chapters 6 and 7) should prevent any milk contamination.

# QUICK TIPS FOR CHAPTER 10

## Breast shield size

- Pain can be caused by using the wrong breast shield size

- Check that your nipple can move freely and is not red or white after pumping

- Measure the diameter of your nipple to find the right breast shield size

- Check size regularly as you may need a different size as your pumping journey continues

## Suction level

- Pumping at too high a suction level can cause pain

- It is also less efficient

- Gradually increase suction until it is uncomfortable and then go back one to find the right level for you

## Yeast infection / thrush

- Nipple and breast pain can be caused by thrush

- Shiny, cracked skin is another sign

- Your doctor can offer treatment for you and your baby

- Pasteurise milk that you pumped while you had thrush to kill the infection before freezing

- Diet and probiotic supplements, and regularly changing breast pads, can help prevent infection

## Nipple vasospasm

- Vasospams are a painful narrowing of blood vessels, often triggered by cold

- Sometimes caused by thrush or damaged nipples, or by Raynaud's Phenomenon

- Avoid the cold: keep warm while pumping and use dry heat on your breasts after pumping

- Take safe painkillers

- Avoid caffeine, nicotine and some medications

- Take a magnesium and /or B6 supplement

## Milk blisters

- Caused by skin growing over the opening of one of your milk ducts

- Treat by applying hot compresses and saline soaks to your nipples

- Remove the skin, or ask your healthcare provider to do it for you

- Massage your breast while pumping to release the blocked milk

- Use painkillers if pumping is painful, but continue to pump regularly

- Tackle oversupply issues and avoid compressing your breasts.

## Clogged ducts

- Ducts can become blocked when they are not drained properly

- You may feel a lump in your breast and it will feel warm and painful to the touch

- Address clogged ducts straight away to avoid mastitis

- Apply a hot compress or soak your breasts before pumping

- Consider pumping in the shower with a manual pump and using a thick comb to massage your breast

- Use breast compressions and massage while pumping

- Pump often and make sure your breasts are fully drained

- Avoid compressing your breasts, tackle oversupply issues, and move your breast shield around while pumping to make sure all of your ducts are being emptied

- Consider taking a lecithin supplement

## Mastitis

- Your breast can become inflamed due to clogged ducts or infection

- As well as pain, you might feel swelling, heat, and flu-like symptoms

- Get plenty of rest, eat and drink well

- Ask for help in caring for your baby so you can concentrate on getting well

- If symptoms are mild and have been present for less than 24 hours, treat as you would a clogged duct

- If symptoms are severe, continue for longer than 24 hours, or are accompanied by clear signs of infection, see your doctor

- Avoid compressing your breasts, tackle oversupply issues, and try to support your immune system with a good diet and enough rest

- Consider taking a lecithin supplement

## Bad back or neck

- Caused by awkward posture during pumping

- Make sure you are sitting comfortably

- Consider using angled breast shields

- Change position while pumping so you don't get stiff

## Dry or cracked nipples

- Use nipple cream, coconut oil, or breastmilk to soothe and moisturise cracked ipples

- Check common causes of nipple pain and the positioning of your nipple in the pump

- Change breast pads regularly and allow your nipples to air dry

- Use coconut oil or nipple cream on your breast shield as lubrication

- Cold compresses can soothe pain, or take safe painkillers

- Small amounts of blood in your milk are fine to give to your baby

- If your milk turns red and it is not from blood, dump it: it is likely infected with bacteria

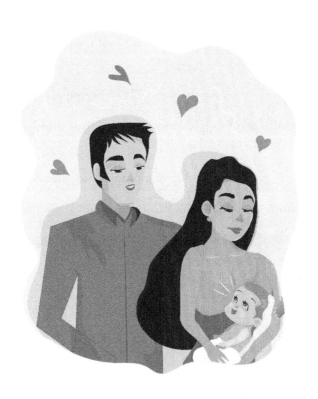

# 11. TROUBLESHOOTING: YOUR BABY

Pumping is only half of the equation when it comes to exclusively pumping; as well as expressing your milk, you also need to actually feed it to your baby. Newborns especially often struggle with digestive issues, and you may encounter problems with bottle-feeding on occasion as well. This chapter looks at the issues that your baby may encounter when bottle-fed with breastmilk (many of which will affect nursing or formula-fed babies too) and will suggest some ways to troubleshoot.

## Bottle-feeding issues

Bottle refusal is less common in babies who have been regularly fed from a bottle from early on – it tends to be more of an issue in babies who have been nursed and are not used to drinking from a bottle. But it can still crop up – some babies will have been taking a bottle perfectly happy for weeks and then decide they don't want to any longer, and others might have issues at the start. Here are some ideas to help you troubleshoot issues with bottle-feeding.

## Check the temperature

Especially if your baby is usually fine drinking from a bottle, if they suddenly refuse a feed, it might be that the milk is not at the right temperature for them. Too hot and it will be painful for them, too cold and they might not like it. Test the temperature with a few drops on the back of your hand and adjust as necessary.

## Offer a taster

Sometimes babies need a bit of tempting to get them to drink. Try rubbing some of your breastmilk on the teat of the bottle before offering it to them so that they know what is on offer and are more likely to accept the feed. Encourage your baby to open their mouth by gently rubbing the teat over their upper lip. Sleepy babies especially may need a bit more tempting before they are ready to latch onto the bottle.

## Style of bottle

Some babies will drink from any bottle you offer them, but others are fussier. Especially if your baby is new to bottle feeding, it may take a few tries before you find a style that they are happy to drink from, which is why it is a good idea to wait until you know your baby will accept the type you have gone for before you invest in loads of them.

## Who is feeding them?

If you are usually the one who feeds your baby and your partner is holding the bottle this time, or vice versa, it may be that they are confused by the change and are reluctant to eat because of it. This can often crop up if your baby is going to a new care giver when you go back to work, which is why most will offer a settling in period. There are two main approaches to helping your baby get used to being fed by someone else – either take yourself fully away so that they don't have the option to default to you, or start the feed yourself and then pass them over once they have started drinking. Hopefully, once they are started, they will be too distracted to stop and will get accustomed to being fed by someone else.

## Make sure they are actually hungry…

Your baby might refuse a feed if they are simply not hungry just then. Look out for hunger cues – rooting, sucking on hands, beginning to fuss – before offering a bottle. These can be difficult to spot in the early days but you will soon get better at recognising your baby's unique cues. If they aren't interested right now, try again when you start to see them acting ready for a feed.

## …but not too hungry

Try to offer milk before your baby becomes too hungry. They often get quite upset when they are very hungry and won't be able to latch onto the bottle. If your baby is too agitated, focus on calming them down, then offer the bottle again. You might need to dribble a little breastmilk slowly into their mouths to get them ready to suck.

## Find a calm place

Babies, especially older babies, can easily be distracted and many won't settle to a feed if there is a lot going on, preferring to pay attention to what is around them. Finding a quiet spot can help them to focus on feeding.

## Consider positioning

Just like nursing babies, bottle-fed babies will have their preferred position for eating in. Some might want to be held as though you were going to nurse, while others will prefer to face outwards so they can drink and still observe what is going on. Experiment with what your baby likes best. It might change depending on how they are feeling – night-time feeds may be more snuggly, while they want to be more upright during daytime feeds. It will also change as your baby gets older – and as they start wanting to hold the bottle themselves.

### Try movement

A reluctant baby can sometimes be encouraged to drink from a bottle if they are walked, rocked, or bounced while the bottle is offered. Usually once you have gotten them drinking, they will let you sit down again, which is a relief for your arms and back.

### Check the teat size

Bottles come with different teat sizes depending on the age of the baby. It can be difficult to tell these apart just by looking but they are usually marked somewhere with the size. Bottle-feeding issues can occur if you are using the wrong teat size – a too large teat will allow the milk to flow more quickly than your baby can cope with, while a too small teat will cause them to become frustrated. If your baby gags or splutters when offered the bottle, that is a sign that the teat is too large for them. On the other hand, if your baby has been drinking well but is now showing signs of frustration – popping on and off the bottle and drinking much slower than they used to – it is likely time to try a bigger teat.

### Frozen milk

Some babies object to the flavour of thawed milk, especially if your milk has high lipase content that can make it taste soapy and unpleasant when frozen. Scalding or pasteurising the milk before freezing it can help with this. Even without high lipase, frozen breastmilk does taste different from fresh and it might take a while for your baby to get used to it. To help them, consider mixing the frozen milk with fresh – starting with a higher amount of fresh and gradually adjusting the proportions until your baby is happily drinking the frozen milk.

### Developmental stages

Babies go through patches where a lot is happening for them all in one go – and these can often be accompanied with sleep regressions and issues feeding. A lot of parents, for example, report issues with bottle feeding around the four to six-week mark, even in a baby who has been happily drinking from a bottle up until then. Usually the refusal is short-term, and the tricks above can help get them comfortable drinking from a bottle again. One helpful guide is the Wonder Weeks app, which can help to predict when your baby is likely to go through one of these developmental leaps.

### Try a different delivery option

Unless you were nursing for some time before switching to exclusively pumping, it is rare for your baby to refuse the bottle forever. But if you have exhausted all the options and your baby's bottle refusal is continuing, try a different way of feeding them. A cup is a common option – even very young babies can learn to drink from an open cup, although it can be a messy process when you first start practicing. Older babies will be learning to drink from a cup anyway once you start introducing solids, so can have breastmilk in a cup as well as water. For tiny babies, a syringe, teaspoon, or dripper might be an option instead.

### Reflux

Sometimes babies will refuse feeds or act fussy and unsettled when fed because they are suffering from reflux. This is when the milk in your baby's stomach travels back up into their oesophagus. It is very common for babies to have mild reflux in the early months and it is usually not too much of a problem, although you may want to keep them upright after a feed to help the milk stay settled in their stomach. Some parents find propping the baby's mattress up as an angle helps if they are spitting up a lot at night.

But for some babies, reflux is more of an issue and can cause pain and discomfort. This is typically a sign of GORD - gastro-oesophageal reflux disease – which is when stomach acid travels back up along with the milk and causes damage to your baby's oesophagus. Symptoms of GORD include a baby who is very fussy after feeds, has slow or no weight gain, spits up very frequently, and struggles to settle, especially lying down. If you suspect your baby might have GORD, speak to your doctor, who can confirm the diagnosis and suggest ways to manage it, which may include medication.

## Baby digestive issues

When your baby is first born, their digestion is still immature. It needs to develop and be populated by good bacteria before it works efficiently – this is part of the reason we don't offer babies solids until they are 6 months old or so. The upshot of this is that many babies suffer from digestive issues, especially in the first three months, as their digestion develops. When you are feeding your baby breastmilk, you may notice that your baby reacts differently to your milk depending on what you had eaten recently when you pumped that feed. Most babies will be fine with your varied diet, but some might exhibit sensitivities when you have eaten certain foods. If your baby is showing signs of digestive discomfort, there are some things you can try:

## Introduce a probiotic

A baby-safe probiotic can work wonders for your baby's digestion by populating your baby's gut with good bacteria. This not only helps with digestion but also strengthens their immune system. Look for a probiotic that contains *Lactobacillus reuteri* (you may see it written as *L. reuteri)* – studies have shown that this bacterial strain is effective in treating colic symptoms in babies that are fed on breastmilk. Some parents report quite dramatic improvements in their babies on starting them on these probiotics. They can usually be found in drop form – you can mix them with your baby's milk or simply use a teaspoon or dropper to drip them into your baby's mouth.

## Eliminate gas issues

Trapped gas can cause problems for your baby. Signs that your baby is struggling include pulling their legs into their chest, discomfort and crying after a feed, lots of burping and farting, lots of spitting up, and disrupted sleep. Gas isn't necessarily a reaction to the content of your milk itself – babies can have gas issues regardless of whether they are nursed, bottle-fed with breastmilk, or bottle fed with formula. Instead it is often caused by an immature digestive system and taking in too much air while feeding.

Introducing a probiotic can help your baby's immature digestive system operate more effectively (see above). You can also try to reduce the amount of air your baby takes in while feeding by making sure you are using a bottle teat that reduces the airflow, feeding your baby in a more upright position, and burping them well during their feed. Stop them feeding every few ounces to burp them, and then burp them well at the end of the feed too. Massaging their tummy in a circular, clockwise direction can release trapped gas, as can peddling their legs in the air as though they were riding a bike, and gently moving their legs over to one side and then the other.

Sometimes you might notice a correlation between what you eat, and your baby's gas issues. If you notice your baby is gassier on some days than others, you might want to start keeping track of what you have eaten each day and mark your expressed milk accordingly. Then you can see if there are any common patterns. If you find a link between a certain food and your baby's issues, think about eliminating that food from your diet – or at least eating it much less often and not using the milk you pump after eating it for your baby.

**Lactose intolerance and cows' milk protein sensitivity**

Lactose intolerance is a commonly suggested when your baby has digestive issues, but the truth is lactose intolerance is comparatively rare in babies. If you have oversupply or have been using leaked milk on its own for feeds, you may find that your baby is suffering from *lactose overload* (rather than intolerance) as a result of foremilk / hindmilk imbalance. This is characterised by a fussy baby and explosive, often green, nappies. See chapter 4 for advice on coping with oversupply and make sure to always mix any milk you collect from leakage with expressed milk before feeding it to your baby. The issue should disappear once your baby's feed is better balanced.

What is more likely than a lactose intolerance, is that your baby has a sensitivity to cows' milk protein. Lactose is found in human breastmilk as well as cows' milk, but there are specific proteins in cow dairy that often cause sensitivity or allergies in babies. As well as fussiness, symptoms of cows' milk sensitivity include diarrhoea or constipation, a stuffy nose, eczema, or hives. If you suspect that your baby has this sensitivity, you can take them to the doctor to confirm, and look at eliminating cows' dairy from your diet. Don't look for lactose free products, since these often still contain the proteins from cows' milk. Opt for items that are marked as being dairy free instead. Fortunately, the rising popularity of veganism means that it is easier than it used to be to find suitable options – but be aware that many babies who are sensitive to cows' milk are also sensitive to soya. Generally speaking, babies grow out of their sensitivity to cows' milk over time and, by the age of three, most can eat dairy without issue.

## Constipation

Constipation is more common in formula-fed babies than those fed on breastmilk and there is a wide range in what is normal for a breastmilk-fed baby. Some will continue to move their bowels several times a day, others might only go once a week. As long as your baby seems happy and comfortable there is nothing to worry about.

But if your baby is acting like they are uncomfortable, their tummy feels hard or swollen, or they seem to be having difficulty in moving their bowels, they may be suffering from constipation. You may see websites that say that babies fed on breastmilk do not get constipated – but this is not true. It is rarer than for formula-fed babies, but still possible.

Check that your baby is getting enough breastmilk, as one cause of constipation is dehydration. Especially if they have been ill or teething, or just going through a fussy patch, they might not have been drinking as much as they should. Consider giving smaller feeds more frequently if your baby is not wanting to drink a lot at each feed – you don't have to change your pumping routine though if you are still getting as much as they need.

As with releasing trapped wind, massage and peddling your baby's legs can encourage their bowels to unblock. Massage their tummy in a clockwise direction, peddle their legs as though they were riding a bike, and gently rock their hips from side to side. Use olive oil or coconut oil for the massage, or you can buy massage oils that are suitable for babies. If there is a baby massage class nearby, you might want to take your baby along to learn more techniques – massage is a lovely bonding technique as well as a way of treating digestive issues.

If your baby is not yet on solids, they shouldn't need extra water or juice, so don't be tempted to give them this for constipation. The advice you might see to give extra water to bottle-fed babies is aimed at formula-fed babies, not babies fed on breastmilk. Your milk has all the fluids your baby needs. Another regularly shared piece of advice is to treat constipation by inserting the tip of a thermometer into your baby's rectum – this can be effective, but there is a risk of hurting your baby. It is not an ideal solution and should not be done regularly.

If your baby regularly suffers from constipation, consult your doctor – they might prescribe a laxative, and may also want to check your baby over in case there is something going on that is causing the issue. You could also start to track your diet and mark expressed milk accordingly, so that you can see any patterns. A sensitivity to cows' milk protein, for example, can cause constipation.

# QUICK TIPS FROM CHAPTER 11

**Bottle-feeding issues**

- Check the temperature of your milk

- Put some breastmilk on the bottle teat and rub it over your baby's top lip

- Try different styles of bottle

- Encourage them to take a bottle from different people by either removing their normal feeder from their hearing and view, or by getting them to start the feed and then passing them to the new person

- Make sure they are hungry, but not too hungry

- Find a calm place

- Try different positions

- Walk, bounce or rock your baby while offering the bottle

- Check the teat size is not too big or too small

- Check the flavour of thawed milk for high lipase. Scald it to eliminate soapiness and mix with fresh milk to get your baby used to the taste

- See if your baby is having a developmental leap

- Try a cup, teaspoon, syringe or dropper instead of a bottle

- Watch out for symptoms of reflux and consult your doctor if your baby shows signs of GORD

**Baby digestive issues**

- Introduce a probiotic to support good digestion

- Eliminate gas issues: burp your baby well, use a bottle that prevents too much air flow, use massage and peddle your baby's legs, see if your diet is causing gas issues

- Watch out for lactose overload caused by foremilk / hindmilk imbalance

- If your baby is sensitive or allergic to cows' milk protein, eliminate dairy from your diet

- Treat constipation by making sure your baby is drinking enough breastmilk, trying massage, and tracking your diet to see if they have any sensitivities

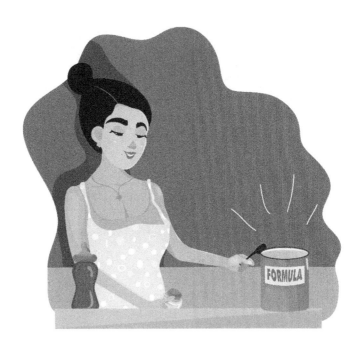

# 12. Combination Feeding

Choosing to exclusively pump is an amazing commitment to your baby's health and wellbeing and shows that you know how good breastmilk is at supporting your baby's development and immune system. But there are times when you might decide to supplement your breastmilk with formula – if you are having issues with low supply, for example, or if you are going back to work, or starting to wean from the pump.

Having made such a commitment to getting breastmilk for your baby, introducing formula might feel strange or wrong. Many babies are fed exclusively on formula and grow up happy and healthy, so try to reassure yourself that your baby will be just fine. Any breastmilk you are able to feed them is a great achievement and supplementing with formula won't take away from that.

## Reasons you might consider supplementing with formula

This is not an exhaustive list, so if your particular reason for wanting to supplement isn't here, that doesn't mean that it is not a valid one. These are some of the common reasons that parents choose to supplement breastmilk with formula when exclusively pumping.

## Low supply

When you are exclusively pumping, you have a much better idea if you are producing enough milk for your baby than if you are nursing, because you can see the difference between how much milk you are pumping and how much your baby is drinking. While you use the tricks and tips in chapter 4 to increase your supply, you may find that you need to supplement with formula to meet your baby's needs. Don't forget to look at pumping efficiency first before you assume your supply is low – it may be that you need to replace parts of your pump or check your suction level and pump positioning before trying to increase supply.

If you are supplementing with formula because your supply is low, but want to continue to express breastmilk for your baby, be sure not to drop pumping sessions just because your baby is not getting breastmilk for that particular feed. Lowering the frequency or length of your pumping sessions will have the effect of decreasing your supply.

## Anxiety and stress

Sometimes the knowledge that your baby is fully reliant on your breastmilk can put a lot of pressure onto your shoulders and make pumping feel stressful. It can also make you feel anxious about whether you will be able to meet your baby's needs. If exclusively pumping to feed your baby is causing anxiety and stress, supplementing with formula can take some of the pressure off. If you know that there is another option available and that your baby will happily accept formula as a substitute, then you can settle into your pumping with less riding on it.

## Returning to work

Depending on how flexible and accommodating your workplace is, and when you return to work, you may find it more of a struggle to pump as much as you need to. Supplementing with formula, as well as using stored breastmilk, can help to make your pumping routine more flexible and diminish any worry that you might not be able to pump enough while at work.

### Your baby needs extra nutrition

On occasion, if your baby had a very low birth weight or is not gaining weight well, your healthcare provider might suggest supplementing your breastmilk with small amounts of formula. As with low supply, make sure to continue to pump regularly even when you are not feeding your baby breastmilk or you risk losing supply.

### You are troubleshooting sleep issues

There is no evidence that supplementing formula actually helps baby sleep longer or not, but it is digested slower than breastmilk, so many people say that giving their baby formula as their last or second-to-last feed before bedtime helped to extend their sleep. Some parents swear by it, others find no difference. There are also lots of different reasons that babies have disrupted nights, not all to do with hunger, so formula is unlikely to help in every instance. If your baby's sleep issues are caused by digestive problems, you probably want to avoid formula at this time of day, since it is harder to digest and more likely to cause problems for your baby.

Try to resist the temptation to use formula at night in place of a middle of the night pumping session, at least while you are still establishing your supply. Night-time pumping sessions are important for increasing and maintaining milk supply, especially in the early months. You can feed your baby formula if you find it helps them sleep better, but still keep the pumping session.

### You are out and about

It's not a good idea to regularly skip pumping sessions and there are usually options if you need to pump out of the house (see chapter 5). But things can happen unexpectedly, so if you are out and don't have breastmilk for your baby (and a one-off nursing session is not an option), you might turn to formula as a stop-gap. You can buy formula ready made-up in chemists and supermarkets.

## You are building a freezer stash

If you are trying to build a freezer stash of breastmilk but don't want to (or can't) add an extra pumping session into your schedule, supplementing with formula can allow you to store milk by replacing one of your baby's feeds.

## You are weaning from pumping

When you decide to stop pumping, you might decide to introduce some formula for your baby alongside the breastmilk you have stored. This will especially be the case if you don't have a big freezer stash and your baby is still young enough to need milk as their main source of nutrients. For baby's over a year, you might skip formula and supplement with cows' milk instead.

## Your milk has a high lipase content

You often don't find out that your milk has the high lipase content that gives it that unpleasant soapy taste when thawed until you have already frozen some feeds. At this point it is too late to try the scalding method, which has to be done before freezing. But the taste might be more easily masked if it is mixed in with formula, which seems to disguise the soapiness better than fresh breastmilk. If your baby will accept the mixture, it saves you from having to dump hard-won milk. It also avoids the pain that comes with mixing the thawed milk with freshly expressed breastmilk, only to find your baby still won't accept it. Dumping formula only hurts your wallet, not your heart!

## You just really, really need a break

We all get to that point at times where the idea of rolling on a bed of broken glass sounds preferable to hooking yourself up to your pump yet again. Check the section on frustration in chapter 9 for help when you feel like this.

Supplementing with formula, either as a one-off or as a regular edition to your schedule, can buy you a little breathing space when pumping feels overwhelming. Keep an eye on your supply just in case of dips, but otherwise embrace the flexibility of combination feeding. Your mental health is more important to your baby than being fed exclusively with breastmilk.

## Times to be wary of supplementing

There are a few situations where you might need to think carefully before introducing formula, because it may do more harm than good. Even with these, it might not be a no, but will need a little extra thought.

## Your baby has GORD

If your baby suffers from this painful form of reflux, supplementing with formula might make the issue worse. Studies have shown that formula-fed babies have more episodes of reflux than babies fed with breastmilk. Because breastmilk is digested more easily, it doesn't sit in your baby's stomach as long, and therefore may be less likely to come back up. If your baby has GORD and you are thinking of introducing formula, speak to your doctor first for recommendations of special formulas you can use.

## Your baby has issues with gas

Breastmilk is easier to digest than formula, so if your baby is suffering from trapped gas, you might want to hold off introducing formula for the moment. For most babies, gas and other digestive issues clear up as they get older, so it may just be a matter of waiting. If you need to supplement with formula, using it earlier in the day and prioritising breastmilk in the afternoon and at night might stop the formula disrupting your baby's night-time sleep.

### Your baby is sensitive to cows' milk protein

Non-dairy formulas do exist, but most contain cows' milk protein and aren't suitable for babies with sensitivities. Annoying though it can be, it might be easier to remove dairy from your own diet than to find a suitable formula. Specialty formulas can also be more expensive. You may be able to get a prescription for a suitable formula though if your baby has allergies.

### Your supply dips

Technically, this is not a reason to not supplement with formula so much as a reason to not drop pumping sessions when you are supplementing with formula. Especially if you pump according to when your baby feeds, rather than on a fixed schedule, you might find your supply dips when you introduce formula. To avoid this issue (unless you are weaning or dealing with oversupply), make sure you are still pumping as much as you were before introducing formula and see chapter 4 for other supply tips.

### Cost

For some families, the cost of formula on top of the outlay already made to purchase pumping equipment might make supplementing with formula undesirable. Breastmilk has the advantage of being free, even if pumps and bottles aren't. If you are on a strict budget, you might need to assess the cost of formula before deciding whether to supplement.

### You don't want to

This may sound obvious – don't supplement with formula if you and your baby are both happy and you are comfortable pumping for every feed. But sometimes the pressure to introduce formula comes from other people, or from the media, rather than from you yourself. Formula does not have any additional nutritional value, your breastmilk is more than adequate to meet your baby's needs. Sleep issues are caused by all sorts of things that have nothing to do with hunger, so if you are being told to introduce formula to address sleep problems, look at other causes and solutions first. Even if your baby is hungry at night, as an exclusive pumper, you have the option that nursing parents don't of simply making a bigger feed up for your baby.

Even if you have low supply and have to supplement with formula for a few weeks, this doesn't have to be a long-term thing if you don't want it to be. Use the tips in chapter 4 to increase your supply and you may well be able to reduce and then stop the formula over time.

## How to supplement breastmilk with formula

Once you decide that supplementing with formula is the right choice for you and your baby, there are three possible ways to go about it. Which to choose will depend on why you are supplementing, how happy your baby is to drink formula, and what works best with your day-to-day routine.

## Option 1: Replace a feed

This is probably the most straight forward. You simply replace one or more of your baby's existing feeds with a bottle of formula. This might be the approach you take especially if you are weaning from the pump, trying to tackle sleep issues, or are returning to work. Choose a feed – perhaps the last or second to last in the day if you are troubleshooting sleep, or one or more middle of the day feeds if you are going back to work – and offer formula for that feed instead of breastmilk. If you are trying to maintain your supply, you will still need to pump to replace that feed but can use the expressed milk later in the day or to start to build a freezer stash. If you are looking to reduce supply, you can drop that feed – either gradually or all at once depending on your propensity to get clogged ducts and how many feeds you are replacing.

This method might not work if your baby is unfamiliar with formula. Some babies are able to switch back and forth without issue, but others take a while to get used to the taste. If your baby is the latter type, you might need to mix feeds at first until they get used to the flavour. See option 3 below. Over time, you can start to change the proportions of breastmilk and formula in the feed until your baby is drinking plain formula.

## Option 2: Top-up a feed

If you are supplementing with formula mainly because of your low supply, or your baby's slow weight gain, feeding them with breastmilk first and then following that feed with a little formula can help to ensure they are getting as much breastmilk as possible. As with option 1, this will only work if your baby is happy to accept plain formula, but you can always start with option 3 and then switch back to topping up feeds as your baby gets used to the taste.

The downside of this method is that it requires you to make up a breastmilk feed *and* a formula feed, which means extra faffing and washing up. With luck though, if you are supplementing while you build your supply, you will only need to use this method for a short amount of time. Enlist help with making feeds and doing the washing up so that you can concentrate on pumping. If budget allows, buying ready made-up formula is more expensive but cuts down on preparation time.

## Option 3: Mix formula and breastmilk

This is the option that often works best if your baby is fussy about accepting formula on its own. It also requires only one bottle, so there is less washing up needed than option 2, although you do still need to prepare both the breastmilk and the formula.

If you are using powdered formula, make up the formula part of the feed in the bottle first to make sure you are getting the correct proportions – use the instructions from the manufacturer on how to make up the feed. Then add breastmilk until you have the right amount. If you are using ready-made formula, you can simply add it to your breastmilk. Swirl the bottle gently to combine them and feed your baby.

If you are using this option because your baby is not keen on the taste of formula, you may need to start with quite a large proportion of breastmilk and a small amount of formula, and adjust the amounts gradually over time.

The downside to this method is that formula cannot be kept for as long as breastmilk. Check the information from the manufacturer and discard any milk within the time given (usually an hour), even if there is more breastmilk in the bottle than formula. To avoid having to throw out breastmilk, you might want to make up smaller feeds at first until you are sure that your baby will accept the mixed feed.

# QUICK TIPS FOR CHAPTER 12

**Reasons you might consider supplementing**

- Low supply

- Anxiety and stress

- Returning to work

- Your baby needs extra nutrition

- You want to see if it will improve their sleep

- You are out and about without breastmilk

- You are building a freezer stash

- You are weaning from pumping

- You want your baby to drink milk with a high lipase content

- You really need a break

**Times to be wary of supplementing**

- Your baby has GORD (severe reflux)

- Your baby has gas issues

- Your baby is sensitive to cows' milk protein

- Your supply dips as a result of supplementing

- Cost of formula

- You are being pressurised by someone else, but don't want to supplement

**How to supplement breastmilk with formula**

- Replace a feed entirely

- Top up a feed by offering breastmilk first and then formula until your baby is full

- Mix the formula and breastmilk in the same feed

- Don't forget; formula needs to be thrown away sooner than breastmilk. If they are combined in the same bottle, it needs to be dumped at the point the formula can no longer be kept, even if there is more breastmilk in the bottle

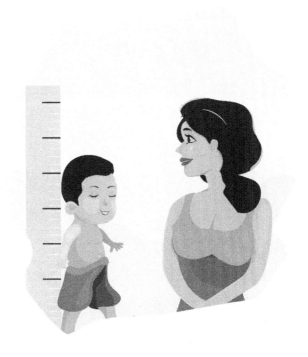

# 13. ENDING YOUR PUMPING JOURNEY

Whether you end up pumping for just a few weeks, or a year or more, at some point it will be time to say goodbye. It can be a surprisingly bitter-sweet time – however pleased you may be to no longer need to pump, it marks the end of one stage of your parenting journey and the beginning of a new one. You may find yourself feeling nostalgic for your early pumping days or even considering your pump with fondness – after all, you have been very reliant on this tool. On the other hand, you may be completely over it and feel more than ready to be done pumping. However, you feel about your pumping journey coming to an end is valid.

Weaning from your pump is a process in its own right and how you decide to go about it will depend on how old your baby is, how often you are currently pumping, what your supply is like, and how prone you are to issues like clogged ducts and mastitis. The good news is that it is likely to be easier to wean from the pump than to stop nursing – your baby is already used to drinking from a bottle and you have likely developed soothing techniques that don't require offering up a breast, so the emotional and practical impact can be a little easier to handle.

## When to wean

There is no right or wrong answer to whether it is the correct time to wean or not. There are lots of factors at play that might make you feel like it is time to be done with pumping. Some people decide to wean once they go back to work, for example, while others will continue for months pumping at work. Some wean at the one-year mark, for others it might be earlier or later. You might have set yourself a goal and be ready to wean now that you have reached it. Or you might make the decision that your family and your mental health will be better off if you are no longer pumping. If your period has returned, it might be harder to meet your baby's needs (milk supply is usually lower during menstruation). Or you might be looking towards your next baby and want to wean because you are pregnant or trying to conceive. Likely there will be a combination of reasons that make you decide that it is the right time for you.

Weaning won't necessarily be an all or nothing process either. You might drop sessions until pumping feels like less of a chore, and then continue with your remaining sessions for a while longer. Or there might be a hard deadline by which you need to have weaned by, such as a medical procedure, which means you need to work out your weaning schedule accordingly.

## Before weaning, decide what you will feed your child

Before you decide to wean from the pump, you also need to decide what to give to your baby instead of freshly expressed milk. If they are over one year-old and well-established on solids, you can offer them cows' milk, but if they are younger and still rely on milk for most of their nutrients, you will need to decide whether you will move them onto formula or try to build a freezer stash so they can continue on breastmilk for longer.

Whatever you choose, if your baby is still a way from their first birthday, you'll need to do some planning before you can start weaning. If you will be moving your baby onto formula and they are not yet used to drinking it, you will want to start introducing it to your baby alongside breastmilk at first, since they may not accept it straight away. Combining formula and breastmilk in each feed can help to acclimatise your baby to the flavour – see chapter 12 for information on introducing formula and combining it with breastmilk.

If you want to continue to offer your baby breastmilk after you have finished pumping, you need to build a freezer stash. This may mean you actually increase the amount you pump at first, in order to get ahead of your baby's needs and have milk to spare for the freezer. Alternatively, you might keep a pumping session in place after your baby drops a feed or give your baby formula for one feed so you can freeze your pumped milk.

To work out how much milk you will need to store, put a ballpark on how long you want your baby to continue to have breastmilk – make sure it is something realistic as you are unlikely to be able to build a big enough stash to keep them going for more than a few months. Multiply the number of days by how many ounces your baby drinks on average in a day and you will know how much milk you need to have stored to reach your goal. You may need to adjust either your goal or your weaning date if this is an unreachable figure, or consider supplementing with formula.

Bear in mind too that milk can go off, even if it is in the freezer – refer to chapter 6 for a reminder of how long you can store milk for. If you have already been freezing your milk, you are ahead of the game. Consider using the frozen milk you already have for feeds so that you can freeze all the fresh milk you are expressing – this will give you the longest amount of time to use the milk in your freezer before it goes off.

## How to wean

How long this process will take depends very much on how many pumping sessions you are currently doing each day and how prone you are to getting clogged ducts. The best approach is to go slowly, dropping one pumping session at a time, rather than trying to stop cold. It is best not to try to drop more than one session a week, which gives your body time to adjust to the changing demand. You can go much more slowly than this too – some people keep the final two sessions for a month or two before finishing altogether.

How you drop each session can vary depending on your preferences. This is very similar to how you would drop a session when your baby's feeding schedule changes (see chapter 5) but the difference is that you won't be adding the time to your other pumping sessions. You can choose to drop a pumping session all in one go, if you tend not to have problems with clogged ducts, or you can go more slowly. If you are going slowly, the options are to gradually reduce the time you pump for, reduce how many ounces you pump, or push the timing of the session back until it is only an hour before the next one, then drop it altogether. If your baby is a bit older and your sessions are already well spaced out, you might find it easier to reduce pumping time or volume instead of moving the session.

You will want to start with dropping your middle of the day pumping sessions instead of the first or last one of the day to avoid engorgement overnight. That said, if you are still pumping in the middle of the night, drop that session first, both to get more sleep and to encourage your body to lower milk production. Once you have dropped one daytime pumping session, move onto the next. You might want to go for non-adjacent sessions to make the process a bit more comfortable. For example, if you were pumping at 6 am, 9 am, 12 pm,

3 pm, 6 pm, and 9 pm you might drop the 9 am and 3 pm feeds first (one at a time) and then the 12 pm and 6 pm ones. If you are down to as few as four pumping sessions, you'll just drop the two in the middle of the day first.

In the scenario above, where you still had 6 pumping sessions a day before starting weaning, you will likely want to bring the final pumping session a bit earlier, so that you are not going more than 12 hours between sessions. Once you are down to only two pumping sessions and your body has adjusted, decide which of the final two sessions to drop first. You might drop the morning one, if this means you can get more sleep or will be able to get out of the house more easily in the morning, or you might drop the evening one if you would prefer to get back the time to do other things at the end of the day.

Once you decide which session you will drop first, start to reduce the time or volume that you pump for that session. It is best not to go cold turkey on a pumping session at this point unless you really need to be done with pumping quickly. You will still do a full pump at the other session. When you have the session you are dropping down to just a few minutes, it is time to stop it altogether. Again, give your body some time to adjust before you start tackling your final session.

Finally, go through the same process for your last remaining pumping session. With luck, you will already be noticing a drop in supply from having ended your other pumping sessions. Again, gradually reduce the time or volume you pump for until you are down to just a few minutes or ounces. Then drop the session. You might need to pump again a few days later, if you are struggling with engorgement – pump just enough to relieve the pressure, rather than aiming for a full session.

And you are done! Time to pack away the pump and celebrate the freedom of no longer needing to be tied to it every day.

## Dealing with engorgement and clogged ducts

As you reduce your sessions, you may find you have issues with engorgement or with clogged ducts that lead to discomfort or pain. This is a normal part of the weaning process, especially if you have dropped a session all at once. If you can, you may want to go more slowly to reduce the discomfort.

The usual remedy for engorgement is to pump, but if you are aiming to reduce your supply, you don't want to encourage your body to keep making milk. If engorgement is getting too uncomfortable, pump just enough to relieve the pain, but stop as soon as you feel more comfortable. Instead of upping your pumping sessions again, you want to use similar tricks to those described in chapter 4 for tackling oversupply. These include using cabbage leaves in your bra, using herbs that reduce supply, or going onto an oestrogen-based birth control.

If you do get a clogged duct while weaning, it is important to tackle it so that you don't risk mastitis. In this case, you might need to temporarily pump or hand express more on the side that has the issue, just until the duct is unblocked. Use massage and hot compresses to get the duct unblocked as quickly as possible. Consider starting on a lecithin supplement to prevent further problems arising, and use other tricks to help reduce your supply, which will also minimise the likelihood of getting clogged ducts.

## Hormones and weaning

You may not notice any changes when you stop pumping, especially if you go slowly and were already down to relatively few pumping sessions per day before you started the weaning process. But as your body stops producing milk, your levels of the hormones involved in breastmilk production – prolactin and oxytocin – will also drop. Since both hormones are involved in feelings of well-being, calmness and love, it makes sense that some people find themselves feeling sad or irritable while weaning, especially when you consider that this is a big step in your parenting journey.

Your hormones will regularise over time, but if you are struggling with the emotions that come with weaning, reach out for help and support. Make sure you continue to have bonding time with your baby – harder to juggle if you have gone back to work, but important to remind yourself that your relationship with your child is much wider than being the provider of their milk. You may also want to slow down the weaning process; the drop in hormones will be more intense the faster you go, so a gradual process is best to allow your body to adjust to the changing hormones as well as to the change in milk supply.

# QUICK TIPS FOR CHAPTER 13

## When to wean

• There are lots of different reasons you might choose to wean

• Only you can decide if it is the right time for you

• It doesn't have to be all or nothing - you can drop some sessions and keep others for a while longer

• Go as fast or slow as you need

## Decide what to feed your child

• Babies who are already over one can get the nutrients they need from solids and cows' milk

• Younger babies will need stored breastmilk or formula

• Start your baby on formula before weaning to make sure they will accept it

• Or build your freezer stash before weaning to make sure you have enough to reach your goal

## How to wean

• Start by dropping one session at a time, one session per week (or slower)

• You can try dropping a session all at once

• Or go gradually by reducing the time or volume you pump, or extending the time between sessions

• Drop daytime feeds first, keeping the ones at the start and end of the day

• Then drop one of the last feeds

- And then drop the final feed
- And celebrate being done!

## Dealing with engorgement and clogged ducts

- Slow down the weaning process to allow your body time to adjust
- To relieve engorgement, pump just enough to feel comfortable and no more
- Try tricks to reduce your supply, such as herbs and cabbage leaves
- Clogged ducts must be dealt with straight away - pump or hand express just on that side
- You can also use massage, breast compressions and hot compresses to clear the blockage
- Start taking a lecithin supplement

## Hormones and weaning

- Weaning can cause a drop in the hormones, prolactin and oxytocin
- This may lead to feelings of sadness or irritability
- Go slowly to reduce the effect
- Reach out for help if you are struggling
- Prioritise bonding time with your baby
- Your hormones will even out over time

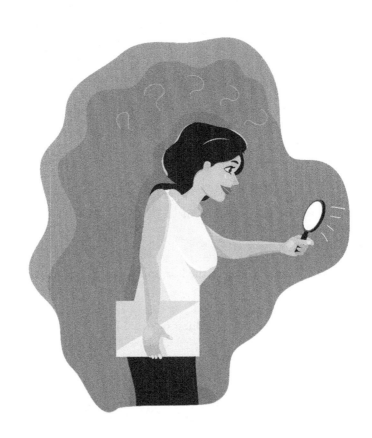

# 14. Finding Support

Like most things, it is easier to find success at exclusive pumping if you have a good support network around you. People who can pick you up when you are feeling down, cheerlead for you when you get frustrated, and celebrate with you when things are going well. Hopefully, you already have some family members or friends who play this role in your life. They might not have experienced exclusively pumping for themselves, but they understand your aims and support you in reaching them.

As well as friends and family, other new parents are a great source of support in the early years. When you have been kept up all night by a teething baby, sharing horror stories with someone who is down there in the parenting trenches with you can make you feel less alone. There's often a great sense of camaraderie among parents who have babies of a similar age. Even if your local parenting groups don't include anyone else who is exclusively pumping, you can find like-minded parents to brighten your day.

Professional support has a role to play too. Although some lactation consultants can be overly focused on nursing, most are open minded and flexible. Doulas specialising in the postpartum period are a growing resource for new mums. And a good counsellor or therapist can provide a professional ear for any mental health issues you encounter.

Finally, online communities are bringing together parents from around the world to support one another, share stories, and give tips and advice. While you might know fewer people in real life (IRL) who have direct experience of exclusively pumping, there are plenty of people online who know exactly what you are going through, because they've been there too.

In this chapter, we'll take a closer look at finding support from these different sources.

## Friends and family

### Your partner

Top of this list should be your partner, if you have one. Even if they aren't genetically related to your baby, your partner is a co-parent and should share in the joys and duties of raising your child, including pumping. While they may not be able to provide milk for your baby, they can support you in many other ways. Sit down with them when you make the decision to exclusively pump and look at how they can best support you, both emotionally and practically. This might be quite an informal chat or, if you are the kind of couple that like to have a solid plan, you could make it more formal. Either way, you need to look at all the other tasks that need to get done through the day – baby care, care for other children, housework, laundry, cooking, food shopping, pets, paid work – and decide who will be responsible for what. Making sure you are on the same page about who is going to take on which tasks can help with avoiding conflict later. Your partner will need to understand that, even if they work outside your home, a lot of your time and mental load will be taken up with pumping, so they will need to do more than their 'fair share' in other areas.

Don't just look at the practicalities when you plan with your partner, but also prepare them for the emotional impact of pumping while caring for a young baby. Suggest ways that you can both have time for yourselves for self-care. Check in with each other regularly and ask your partner to let you know if they have any worries about your mental health, or their own.

## Friends or family members

Whether you have a supportive partner or not, there is a lot that friends and family can do to help out. Family doesn't need to mean blood relatives either, many of us have 'found families' made up of close friends. Those who already have children know a bit about what you are going through and might be able to see when a helping hand is needed without having to be asked. But often your family and friends need a bit more of a nudge.

Asking for help can feel alien when we are so used to being self-sufficient. But becoming a parent is often the moment when we realise how much we need our communities. Don't be afraid to ask for help – just be ready to return the favour someday. Make your request as specific as you can – people generally do want to assist, but don't always know how. Could your friends organise a meal train for you so that you don't have to worry about cooking while you are settling into your pumping routine? Perhaps they could take older children out for you, walk your dog, or hold the baby for an hour so that you can pump (or nap). Or maybe they can meet you for a coffee and give you a chance to talk to another grown up for a while.

Beware of anyone who tries to make you feel guilty about your pumping – it is normal for people to have questions at first, but if there is anyone who regularly suggests that you should be doing something differently, they are not the person to call on for support. They might be a fantastic person normally, but right now you need people who are fully in your corner. Tell them that you are not interested in discussing pumping with them and, if they persist, be ready to take a break from their company for a little while. This can be harder if it is a family member, so call on other family members and your partner for back up at family gatherings if needed. Politely refusing to discuss it and changing the topic if it comes up works for most people, although you might need to do it a few times before they get the message.

## Parenting groups

There are lots of groups out there for new parents. Some are activity-based, such as baby massage, yoga, or music classes, while others are focused on advice and support. Generally, they are a good excuse to get out of the house, eat biscuits, and offload with other parents who are feeling similarly sleep-deprived, lost, and overwhelmed.

## Prenatal groups

You might have been a member of a prenatal group before your baby was even born. Often these groups come together to learn about birth and early parenting, but it is a good idea to keep up with other families once your baby arrives too, especially since they are likely to have had a baby at around the same time. Because you met before your baby arrived, you'll see how differently everyone's journey goes, which can be reassuring.

## Mothers' groups

Often you will be assigned to a mothers' group by the hospital when you give birth, linking you to other parents in the area who have babies of a similar age. Of course, having given birth at around the same time is no guarantee that you will get on with the people in your group, but it is an easy way to get to know other new parents. It is also a good way to find people who are up for outings and understand the need to spend an entire coffee date pumping or juggling a crying baby.

## Breastfeeding groups

These general groups are great for meeting other parents, but there are times when you need specific advice. Although breastfeeding support groups often focus on nursing, most welcome exclusively pumping parents too. Worries about supply, clogged ducts, and engorgement apply whether you are pumping or nursing, so you will likely find you have quite a lot in common with other breastfeeding parents. The Australian Breastfeeding Association can help you find a group near you: https://www.breastfeeding.asn.au/contacts/groups

## Activity groups

With luck, these groups will be a great source of support. But if you are finding that one group or other is too fixated on nursing and makes you feel uncomfortable for pumping instead, it might be better to find a parent group that focuses on a specific activity. Look out for groups teaching baby yoga or massage, or ones focused on sensory play or music and rhyme. Because these groups are structured around the activity, there is less general chat, but you can still get to know other parents, have fun with your baby, and get out of the house. Sometimes not focusing on pumping for a little while can do wonders for your mental health.

## Professional help

Peer support from other new parents is excellent for building a parenting community, but sometimes you need professional help from someone who has training in the particular area that is causing you issues.

## Breastfeeding counsellors

Breastfeeding support groups are usually run by volunteer counsellors. While these aren't paid professionals, they have undergone training to support you in your breastfeeding journey. Ideally, that will include pumping advice but be aware this can be a little hit-and-miss depending on the individual counsellor. You can attend a breastfeeding support group to speak to your local counsellor and some also do home visits. As well as the Australian Breastfeeding Association, La Leche League Australia has counsellors in some areas: http://lllaustralia.org/contact-a-leader-in-your-area/

**Lactation consultants**

Unlike breastfeeding counsellors, lactation consultants are certified professionals and experts in everything to do with lactation. You may have seen one during the early days if you were troubleshooting nursing issues. If you are having difficulties with supply or are regularly coming down with clogged ducts or mastitis, you can talk to a lactation consultant. To avoid any confusion, explain straight away that you are pumping rather than nursing and make it clear that you don't want to revisit the nursing issues (unless you do, of course). Your GP might be able to refer you, or you can find a lactation consultant via the Lactation Consultants of Australia and New Zealand (LCANZ): https://www.lcanz.org/resources/clients/how-do-i-access-a-lactation-consultant/

**Postpartum doulas**

You might be more familiar with doulas providing support during labour and birth, but a growing number of doulas also work with families in the postnatal period. When you are getting used to having a newborn and also needing to pump, having someone on hand to give you calm and caring support can be invaluable. It does come with a cost, however, so factor that into your plans.

Personal recommendations can be useful in finding a good doula, as it is quite a personal relationship. Alternatively, the Find a Doula website can help in finding postnatal doulas near you: https://findadoula.com.au/. When you speak to them, make your pumping part of the conversation so that you can be sure the person you choose will be supportive.

## Therapists or counsellors

If you are struggling with the emotional aspects of pumping, seeking help from a therapist or counsellor is a powerful way to look after your mental health. Some practitioners specialise in new parents, so you may want to look for someone with experience in this area. Your GP might be able to refer you, or you can find an accredited counsellor through the Australian Counselling Association: https://www.theaca.net.au/find-registered-counsellor.php. For short-term help, PANDA's helpline and other resources can get you started: https://www.panda.org.au/.

## Online communities

Whatever else you might say about the internet, it is a fantastic way to find specific communities that you might not have access to in real life. Because exclusive pumping is less well-known as a feeding route than nursing or formula-feeding, there are fewer resources online for pumping parents, but those that exist are very supportive. However good your in-person network may be, sometimes it is a relief to speak to others who are going through the same things as you.

## Social media sites

Facebook especially is full of all sorts of parenting groups and there are a number dedicated to exclusively pumping. Search for exclusive pumping on Facebook to find groups. Not all are active, so check the date of the last post before joining. Or you could even start your own.

Instagram doesn't lend itself as well to the group model, but there are some exclusive pumping accounts that are worth following for tips, ticks, and stories. Some hashtags to look out for are #exclusivepumping, #exclusivelypumping, #exclusivepumpers, #pumpingmom,

#pumpingmoms, #pumprules, #pumpingmilk, #breastpump, #exclusivepumpingmama, and #pumpingmama.

**Forum sites**

Parenting forums can be a good way to find other pumping parents to share stories and exchange advice. It can take a while to get used to the acronyms if you have never used one of these forums before. Some common ones you might see:

- EP/EPing/EPer – the EP stands for exclusive pumping

- DS/DD/DP – dear son, dear daughter, and dear partner. DS or DD might be accompanied by a number which indicates either the birth order or their age, depending on the context

- MOTN – middle of the night

- PP – postpartum

- PPD – pumps per day

- FTM – first time mum

- LO – little one

- EBF – exclusively breastfeeding

- IRL – in real life

BubHub is one forum that is specific to Australia: https://www.bubhub.com.au/community/forums/forum.php. They don't have a dedicated board for exclusive pumpers, but questions are often posted in the breastfeeding support board. Just be aware that you might get comments from parents who don't exclusively pump themselves. For more specific exclusive pumping chat, the American site, What to Expect, has an active exclusive pumping forum: https://community.whattoexpect.com/forums/exclusive-pumping.html

## Family and friends

- If you have a partner, they need to be fully involved

- Make a plan so you are both clear on who is responsible for which chores

- Make time for self-care for both you and your partner

- Friends or family members can be a great help

- Ask for help, don't wait for them to offer

- Be as specific as possible about what you need

- Avoid those who don't support you on your pumping journey, or refuse to discuss it with them

## Parenting groups

- Prenatal groups went through pregnancy with you and can be a source of support after birth too

- Mothers' groups are a good way to meet other new parents

- Breastfeeding groups can support you with specific advice and should be open to pumpers as well as nursing parents

- Groups based around activities can take the focus off feeding and be bonding for you and your baby

## Professional help

- Breastfeeding counsellors are volunteers who can give advice on pumping issues

- Lactation consultants are trained professionals who can advise on problems with supply and mastitis

- Postpartum doulas provide in-home support to new parents

- A counsellor or therapist helps you to look after your mental health

**Online communities**

- Exclusive pumping communities can be found on social media sites such as Facebook or Instagram

- Forum sites allow you to ask specific questions and find other exclusively pumping parents

# CONCLUSION

You've made it to the end, congratulations! You should be well-set up now with all the knowledge you need for a successful exclusively pumping journey. Of course, there will be times when you need some sections of this book more than others, so I hope you will dip in and out as needed to find the advice and troubleshooting you need. Don't forget to use the quick tips at the end of each chapter when you need an easy way to jog your memory.

If nothing else, I hope you have taken away the core message of this book – choosing to exclusively pump breastmilk for your baby is an amazing thing to do. No matter if you do it for a few weeks or over a year, you have made a true commitment to the health and wellbeing of your baby. The journey won't always be smooth, and it may feel lonely at times, so take the time to feel proud of yourself and everything you achieve. One day, this time in your life will be a distant memory. I hope you will look back and know what a fantastic parent you are to have gone above and beyond for your child.

**Further reading and resources**

Although the aim of this guide is to be a comprehensive resource for all your exclusive pumping queries, it is never a bad idea to read more into the topic. As we discussed in chapter 1, arming yourself with information is the best thing you can do to put yourself on the road to success. There are references for every chapter that you can use to find articles about specific topics. In addition, the following resources are good places for further reading:

**Exclusive Pumping blog:** https://exclusivepumping.com/

Written by American mum of three, Amanda Glenn, the exclusive pumping blog has everything from pump reviews to advice on weaning. Amanda, who is a certified lactation counsellor as well as an experienced exclusive pumper, is relatively quick to respond to comments and runs an associated Facebook group and Instagram page.

Amanda also has two short eBooks; *Exclusive Pumping and Milk Supply* and *Weaning from the Pump*. And she has printables and a free five-day email course that you may find helpful. Bear in mind that advice and pump recommendations will be from a US perspective – not all the pump models mentioned on the site are easily available in Australia.

**The Australian Breastfeeding Association:**
https://www.breastfeeding.asn.au/

Champions of everything breastfeeding in Australia, the Australian Breastfeeding Association (ABA) have articles and free pamphlets to cover most breastfeeding concerns, including exclusively pumping. They also hire out hospital grade breast pumps, and their trained volunteers run breastfeeding support groups around the country. In particular, the ABA have a range of resources and advice for those returning to work and are campaigning for more workplaces to become accredited as breastfeeding friendly. For country-specific advice, they are a great port of call.

**KellyMom:** https://kellymom.com/

If you have ever googled anything to do with breastfeeding, you'll likely end up on the KellyMom website sooner or later. This long running site is the brainchild of Kelly Bonyata, an international board certified lactation consultant, who has been working with parents since 1997. The advice on her site is written mainly by Kelly, but with other contributors weighing in too.

Articles are well-researched, authoritative, and based on scientific evidence. The site includes articles aimed specifically at exclusive pumping parents, as well as general tips and advice covering everything from supply to allergies to mastitis. Its no-nonsense approach is excellent for when you want to get straight to the facts.

**La Leche League International:** https://www.llli.org/

La Leche League is an organisation that works around the world to support breastfeeding, including exclusively pumping parents. There are individual branches for each of the countries they work in, but the international site has the most comprehensive collection of articles and advice. Their A-Z of breastfeeding is useful when you want to know more about a particular topic. Although articles about pumping are more focused on nursing parents, there are helpful guides to things like cleaning your pump, storing milk, and issues like allergies, reflux, and GORD (or GERD, as they have it).

# REFERENCES

**Chapter 1**

Reasons to exclusively pump, from Exclusive Pumping:
https://exclusivepumping.com/exclusively-pumping-guide/

How to make a DIY pumping bra, from Nicole Burt Blog:
https://nicoleburtblog.com/diy-pumping-bra/#:~:text=%20DIY%20Pumping%20Bra%20Instructions%3A%20%201%20Buy,wo%20rk%20%28or%20drive%20home%20%29%20More%20, consulted 03/10/2020

Different styles of hands-free bras, from Exclusive Pumping:
https://exclusivepumping.com/best-hands-free-pumping-bras/, consulted 03/10/2020

Article on foremilk / hindmilk, from La Leche League International:
https://www.llli.org/breastfeeding-info/foremilk-and-hindmilk/, consulted 03/10/2020

Best lactation massagers, from the Baby Swag: https://thebabyswag.com/best-lactation-massagers/, consulted 03/10/2020

**Chapter 2**

Best pumps for exclusive pumpers, from Exclusive Pumping:
https://exclusivepumping.com/best-breast-pumps-for-exclusive-pumpers/ consulted 03/10/3030

Open vs closed system pumps, from Breast Pumps Direct:
https://www.breastpumpsdirect.com/open_system_breastpumps_vs_closed_system_breastpumps_a/147.htm#:~:text=The%20difference%20between%20these%20two%20pu

mp%20types%20is,problems%2C%20including%20contamination%20of%20your%20precious%20breast%20milk. consulted 03/10/2020

Buying second hand, from Spectra: https://spectra-baby.com.au/buying-second-hand-breast-pump/, consulted 04/10/2020

Replacing parts, from Pumping Mamas: https://pumpingmamas.com/replace-breast-pump-parts/, consulted 04/10/2020

Breast pump parts, from Pumping Mamas: https://pumpingmamas.com/breast-pump-parts/, consulted 04/10/2020

Chapter 3

Colostrum, from La Leche League International: https://www.llli.org/breastfeeding-info/colostrum-general/, consulted 04/10/2020

Expressing colostrum, from La Leche League International: https://www.llli.org/breastfeeding-info/colostrum-prenatal-antenatal-expression/, consulted 04/10/2020

Letdowns, from Exclusive Pumping: https://exclusivepumping.com/how-to-boost-milk-supply-letdowns/, consulted 04/10/2020

Breastfeeding hormones, from Breastfeeding Problems: https://www.breastfeeding-problems.com/breastfeeding-hormones.html, consulted 04/10/2020

Prolactin and breastfeeding, from Very Well Family: https://www.verywellfamily.com/prolactin-and-breastfeeding-3860902, consulted 04/10/2020

Expressing for a new-born, from Exclusive Pumping: https://exclusivepumping.com/exclusive-pumping-for-a-newborn/, consulted 04/10/2020

Chapter 4

When does supply regulate, from Exclusively Pumping: https://exclusivepumping.com/when-is-milk-supply-established/, consulted 04/10/2020

Breast milk oversupply, from Undefining Motherhood: https://undefiningmotherhood.com/breast-milk-oversupply/, consulted 04/10/2020

Over and undersupply of breast milk, from Pediatric Partners: https://pediatricpartners.blogspot.com/2016/09/over-and-under-supply-of-breast-milk.html, consulted 04/10/2020

Does drinking water affect breastfeeding, from Very Well Family: https://www.verywellfamily.com/does-drinking-more-water-affect-breastfeeding-284285, consulted 04/10/2020

Increasing milk supply, from Exclusively Pumping: https://exclusivepumping.com/increasing-milk-supply/, consulted 04/10/2020

Power pumping, from Healthline: https://www.healthline.com/health/breastfeeding/power-pumping, consulted 04/10/2020

Oatmeal for increasing milk supply, From Kelly Mom: https://kellymom.com/bf/got-milk/supply-worries/oatmeal/, consulted 05/10/2020

Motilium (domperidone) for breastfeeding, from BellyBelly, https://www.bellybelly.com.au/breastfeeding/motilium-domperidone-for-breastfeeding/, consulted 05/10/2020

Drugs affecting milk supply during lactation, from NPS Medicinewise: https://www.nps.org.au/australian-prescriber/articles/drugs-affecting-milk-supply-during-lactation, consulted 05/10/2020

Find a consultant, from LCANZ: https://www.lcanz.org/find-a-lactation-consultant/, consulted 05/10/2020

Oversupply – gift or curse? From La Leche League International: https://www.llli.org/oversupply-gift-curse/, consulted 06/10/2020

Lecithin use while breastfeeding, from Drugs.com: https://www.drugs.com/breastfeeding/lecithin.html, consulted 06/10/2020

Cabbage leaves for breast engorgement, from Babyology: https://babyology.com.au/baby/feeding/breastfeeding/cabbage-leaves-for-breast-engorgement-relief-fact-or-fiction/, consulted 06/10/2020

Sage and other herbs for decreasing milk supply, from Kelly Mom https://kellymom.com/bf/can-i-breastfeed/herbs/herbs-oversupply/, consulted 06/10/2020

Chapter 5

Pumping at night, from Love our Littles: https://loveourlittles.com/pumping-at-night/, consulted 05/10/2020

Exclusive pumping for a newborn, from Exclusive Pumping: https://exclusivepumping.com/exclusive-pumping-for-a-newborn/, consulted 06/10/2020

How much expressed milk will my baby need? From Kelly Mom: https://kellymom.com/bf/pumpingmoms/pumping/milkcalc/, consulted 07/10/2020

Calculating how much breastmilk to put in a bottle, from Very Well Family https://www.verywellfamily.com/how-much-breast-milk-should-i-put-in-a-bottle-431802, consulted 07/10/2020

How to drop middle of the night pumping sessions in 4 steps, from Exclusively Pumping, https://exclusivepumping.com/drop-middle-of-the-night-pumping-sessions/, consulted 07/10/2020

How to stop pumping, from Working Mother: https://www.workingmother.com/momlife/13590156/how-to-stop-pumping/, consulted 07/10/2020

What to feed your baby, from NHS UK: https://www.nhs.uk/start4life/weaning/what-to-feed-your-baby/10-12-months/#anchor-tabs

Breastfeeding in public - your legal rights, from Australian Breastfeeding Association: https://www.breastfeeding.asn.au/bf-info/breastfeeding-and-law/legalright, consulted 07/10/2020

Is it illegal to eat and drive? From Law Path: https://lawpath.com.au/blog/is-it-illegal-to-eat-and-drive, consulted 07/10/2020

How to pump breast milk while caring for your baby, from Exclusively Pumping: https://exclusivepumping.com/pump-and-take-care-of-a-baby-at-the-same-time/, consulted 07/10/2020

**Chapter 6**

Storing human milk, from La Leche League International: https://www.llli.org/breastfeeding-info/storingmilk/, consulted 09/10/2020

Hands, A. Variations in recommendations for storing expressed breast milk, from the Breastfeeding Network: https://www.breastfeedingnetwork.org.uk/breastfeeding-help/expressing-storing/variations-in-recommendations-for-storing-expressed-breast-milk/, consulted 09/10/2020

How long can milk really sit out before it goes bad? From Mom Tricks: https://www.momtricks.com/breastfeeding/how-long-can-breast-milk-sit-out/, consulted 09/10/2020

**Chapter 7**

How to keep your breast pump kit clean: The essentials, from Centers for Disease Control and Prevention:

https://www.cdc.gov/healthywater/hygiene/healthychildcare/infantfeeding/breastpump.html, consulted 13/10/2020

4 steps to quickly dry breast pump parts at work (plus 3 bonus tips), from Pumping Mamas, https://pumpingmamas.com/how-to-quickly-dry-breast-pump-parts-at-work/, consulted 13/10/2020

8 tips for washing baby bottles and breast pump parts, from Exclusively Pumping: https://exclusivepumping.com/washing-baby-bottles-breast-pump-parts/, consulted 13/10/2020

Sterilising bottle-feeding equipment, from Baby Center: https://www.babycenter.com.au/a554982/sterilising-bottle-feeding-equipment, consulted 13/10/2020

**Chapter 8**

*Breastfeeding and Work: Your Rights at Work* (2017), from the Australian Breastfeeding Association

Employers, from the Australian Breastfeeding Association: https://www.breastfeeding.asn.au/workplace/employers, consulted 14/10/2020

Workplace discrimination, from the Fair Work Ombudsman: https://www.fairwork.gov.au/how-we-will-help/templates-and-guides/fact-sheets/rights-and-obligations/workplace-discrimination, consulted 18/10/2020

*Breastfeeding and Childcare: Important information for parents* (2014), from the Australian Breastfeeding Association

**Chapter 9**

Beaver, D. (2019), The Life/Death/Life Cycle of the Exclusive Pumping Journey, from Medium: https://medium.com/@drbeaver/the-life-death-life-cycle-of-the-exclusive-pumping-journey-136513f8bf69, consulted 20/10/2020

Borra, C., Iacovou, M. & Sevilla, A. (2015) New Evidence on Breastfeeding and Postpartum Depression: The Importance of Understanding Women's Intentions. *Maternal Child Health Journal* 19, 897–907

Levine, H. (2020), Breastfeeding With Dysphoric Milk Ejection Reflex (D-MER), from What to Expect: https://www.whattoexpect.com/first-year/breastfeeding/dysphoric-milk-ejection-reflex/, consulted 22/10/2020

Forward, J. (2020), Postpartum depression expert explains birth trauma, from CHRON: https://www.chron.com/neighborhood/woodlands/article/Postpartum-depression-expert-explains-birth-trauma-15660966.php, consulted 22/10/2020

Watkins S, Meltzer-Brody S, Zolnoun D, Stuebe A. (2011) Early breastfeeding experiences and postpartum depression. *Obstetrics and Gynaecology,* 118(2 Pt 1):214-21

Wells, S., To the exclusively pumping mama: A note of encouragement, from Motherly, https://www.mother.ly/life/to-the-exclusively-pumping-mama, consulted 20/10/2020

Self-care for anxiety, from MIND UK: https://www.mind.org.uk/information-support/types-of-mental-health-problems/anxiety-and-panic-attacks/self-care-for-anxiety/#collapsef7731, consulted 21/10/2020

PANDA: https://www.panda.org.au/, consulted 21/10/2020

What is Dysphoric Milk Ejection Reflex? From D-MER.org: https://d-mer.org/, consulted 22/10/2020

**Chapter 10**

Guide to Choosing the Right Breast Shield Size, from Milkbar: https://milkbarbreastpumps.com.au/blogs/news/guide-to-choosing-the-right-breast-shield-size, consulted 22/10/2020

Is pumping causing you pain? From Motherlove, https://www.motherlove.com/blogs/all/is-pumping-causing-you-pain, consulted 22/10/2020

Kent, J. C., L. R. Mitoulas, M. D. Cregan, D. T. Geddes, M. Larsson, D. A. Doherty, and P. E. Hartmann. (2008) Importance of Vacuum for Breastmilk Expression, *Breastfeeding Medicine,* 11-19

Another Breast Pumping Mystery Solved! Does Higher Pump Suction Mean More Milk?, from Medela Australia: https://www.medela.com.au/breastfeeding/blog/breast-milk-expressing-tips/another-breast-pumping-mystery-solved-higher-pump-suction-mean-milk, consulted 22/10/2020

How to pasteurise breastmilk, from Breastfeeding Moms Unite, http://www.breastfeedingmomsunite.com/how-to-pasteurize-breast-milk/, consulted 22/10/2020

A pain in the boob: breastfeeding and thrush, from Exclusive Pumping, https://exclusivepumping.com/breastfeeding-thrush/, consulted 22/10/2020

Nipple blanching and vasospasm, from KellyMom: https://kellymom.com/bf/concerns/mother/nipple-blanching/, consulted 24/10/2020

Medicines and breastfeeding, from Health Direct: https://www.healthdirect.gov.au/medicines-and-breastfeeding, consulted 24/10/2020

Vasospams, from International Breastfeeding Centre: https://ibconline.ca/information-sheets/vasospasm/, consulted 24/10/2020

How to treat a milk blister when you are exclusively pumping, from Exclusive Pumping: https://exclusivepumping.com/milk-blister/, consulted 24/10/2020

How do you treat a milk blister?, from KellyMom: https://kellymom.com/bf/concerns/mother/nipplebleb/, consulted 24/10/2020

Best nipple creams for breastfeeding moms, from Exclusive Pumping: https://exclusivepumping.com/best-nipple-creams/, consulted 24/10/2020

Managing blocked milk ducts and treating mastitis, from Medela: https://www.medela.us/breastfeeding/articles/managing-blocked-milk-ducts-and-treating-mastitis, consulted 24/10/2020

Lecithin treatment for recurrent plugged ducts, from KellyMom: https://kellymom.com/bf/concerns/mother/lecithin/, consulted 24/10/2020

Plugged ducts and mastitis, from KellyMom: https://kellymom.com/bf/concerns/mother/mastitis/, consulted 24/10/2020

A pain in the boob: clogged milk ducts and how to clear them, from Exclusive Pumping: https://exclusivepumping.com/clogged-ducts/, consulted 24/10/2020

Recurrent mastitis or plugged ducts, from Kelly Mom, https://kellymom.com/bf/concerns/mother/recurrent-mastitis/, consulted 24/10/2020

A pain in the boob: preventing and treating mastitis, from Exclusive Pumping: https://exclusivepumping.com/a-pain-in-the-boob-mastitis/, consulted 24/10/2020

Red milk: what causes your milk to turn red? From Infant Risk: https://www.infantrisk.com/content/red-milk-what-causes-your-milk-turn-red, consulted 24/10/2020

Cracked and bleeding nipples when pumping breastmilk, from Exclusive Pumping: https://exclusivepumping.com/bleeding-nipples-when-pumping/, consulted 24/10/2020

**Chapter 11**

Bottle refusal, from Institute for the Advancement of Breastfeeding & Lactation Education, https://lacted.org/iable-breastfeeding-education-handouts/bottle-refusal/, consulted 24/10/2020

Hunger cues, from KellyMom, https://kellymom.com/bf/normal/hunger-cues/, consulted 24/10/2020

Bottles and other tools, from La Leche League International, https://www.llli.org/breastfeeding-info/bottles/, consulted 24/10/2020

Sung, V., F. D'Amico, M.l D. Cabana, K. Chau, G. Koren, F. Savino, H. Szajewska, G. Deshpande, C. Dupont, F. Indrio, S. Mentula, A. Partty, D. Tancredi (2018), Lactobacillus reuteri to Treat Infant Colic: A Meta-analysis, *Pediatrics* 141 (1)

10 ways to soothe baby's gas pain, from Breastfeeding Problems, https://www.breastfeeding-problems.com/baby-gas-pain.html, consulted 24/10/2020

Dairy and other food sensitivities in breastfed babies, from KellyMom, https://kellymom.com/health/baby-health/food-sensitivity/, consulted 24/10/2020

Breastfeeding challenges: constipation, from NHS UK, https://www.nhs.uk/start4life/baby/breastfeeding/breastfeeding-challenges/constipation/, consulted 25/10/2020

Reflux (GOR) and GORD, from the Royal Children's Hospital Melbourne: https://www.rch.org.au/kidsinfo/fact_sheets/Reflux_GOR/, consulted 25/10/2020

**Chapter 12**

Mixed feeding: supplementing breastfeeding with formula, from Raising Children, https://raisingchildren.net.au/newborns/breastfeeding-bottle-feeding/bottle-feeding/mixed-feeding, consulted 25/10/2020

Will giving formula or solids at night help baby to sleep better? From KellyMom, https://kellymom.com/nutrition/starting-solids/solids-sleep/, consulted 25/10/2020

How to get baby to drink high lipase breastmilk, from Exclusive Pumping, https://exclusivepumping.com/high-lipase-breastmilk/, consulted 25/10/2020

I think my baby's got reflux, from La Leche League GB, https://www.laleche.org.uk/i-think-babys-got-reflux/, consulted 25/10/2020

Supplementing breastmilk with formula, from Exclusive Pumping, https://exclusivepumping.com/supplementing-with-formula/, consulted 25/10/2020

**Chapter 13**

How to wean from the pump when you are exclusively pumping, from Exclusive Pumping: https://exclusivepumping.com/weaning-from-the-pump/, consulted 25/10/2020

Weaning from the pump, from KellyMom: https://kellymom.com/bf/pumpingmoms/pumping/weaning-from-pump/, consulted 25/10/2020

Sadness and depression during (and after) weaning, from KellyMom, https://kellymom.com/ages/weaning/wean-how/depression-and-weaning/, consulted 25/10/2020

**Chapter 14**

The hidden benefits of mothers' groups, from Medibank: https://www.medibank.com.au/livebetter/families/new-parents/the-hidden-benefits-of-mothers-groups/, consulted 27/10/2020

Local support groups, from the Australian Breastfeeding Association: https://www.breastfeeding.asn.au/contacts/groups, consulted 27/10/2020

Contact a leader in your area, from La Leche League Australia: http://lllaustralia.org/contact-a-leader-in-your-area/, consulted 27/10/2020

How do I access a lactation consultant? From LCANZ: https://www.lcanz.org/resources/clients/how-do-i-access-a-lactation-consultant/, consulted 27/10/2020

Find a doula, https://findadoula.com.au/, consulted 27/10/2020

PANDA, https://www.panda.org.au/, consulted 27/10/2020

Find a registered counsellor, from the Australian Counselling Association: https://www.theaca.net.au/find-registered-counsellor.php, consulted 27/10/2020

BubHub: https://www.bubhub.com.au/community/forums/forum.php, consulted 27/10/2020

Exclusive pumping, from What to Expect: https://community.whattoexpect.com/forums/exclusive-pumping.html, consulted 27/10/2020

Made in the USA
Monee, IL
08 July 2023

38870444R00109